HERPES
DISEASES
and your health

HERPES DISEASES
and your health

by
Henry H. Balfour, Jr., M.D.
and Ralph C. Heussner

University of Minnesota ▪ Minneapolis

Publication of this book was assisted
by a grant from the McKnight Foundation
to the University of Minnesota Press's program
in the health sciences.

Published by the University of Minnesota Press,
2037 University Avenue Southeast, Minneapolis MN 55414

Printed in the United States of America
Designed by Gale L. Houdek
Cover photo by Liz Harrison

Library of Congress Cataloging in Publication Data

Balfour, Henry H.
  Herpes diseases and your health.

  Bibliography: p.
  Includes index.
  1. Herpesvirus diseases. 2. Health. I. Heussner,
Ralph C. II. Title.
RC147.H6B34 1984   616.9'25   84-7514
ISBN 0-8166-1335-4

The University of Minnesota is an equal-opportunity educator
and employer.

For
Carol L. Balfour
and
Virginia Mae Heussner

Contents

Preface / ix

If Vietnam was the first television war, herpes is the first television epidemic. Newspapers, magazines, and television have played a role in alerting the public to the extensive spread of genital herpes and the need for prevention and treatment. Now everyone has heard of herpes. But herpes is more than a venereal disease. In fact, herpes belongs to a family of five closely related viruses that cause such common and varied conditions as chickenpox, cold sores, shingles, and mono.

Why should *you* read this book? Because you almost certainly have one of the five human herpesviruses in your own body right now, and you should know what that means. Herpes is short for herpes simplex virus—of which there are two types, both capable of causing genital herpes. But there are three other herpesviruses you should learn about because they may be more important to you than herpes simplex.

Why did I write this book? My Clinical Virology Service at the University of Minnesota has studied hundreds of patients with infections due to all five members of the herpes family. By investigating ways of tipping the balance in favor of the patient rather than the virus, our research team has learned what to expect in the typical case as well as the extreme. For example, many of our patients have weakened immunity due to cancer or drugs that protect a transplanted organ. With only part of their immune defenses intact, such "immunosuppressed" patients are easy prey for the herpesviruses. But we have even found methods of prevention and treatment of herpes infections in these patients. Our experience has enabled us to appreciate the entire spectrum of herpesvirus diseases. Sharing that perspective will give you the knowledge to overcome your concerns about herpes.

There are too many misconceptions about herpesviruses, and I want to set the record straight in this book. Some of these misconceptions are due to incomplete news reporting. Television and newspapers are so crowded with features about daily events that only a smidgen of the herpes story ever reaches you. Even the latest herpes books written for the public are often incomplete and sometimes inaccurate. Clearly, the whole truth about herpes should be told and told so that you can understand it. In order to do just that, I collaborated with Ralph Heussner, a former reporter and editor at the *Atlanta Journal* who now serves as the Chief Public Information Officer for the University of Minnesota Health Sciences Center. Although Ralph and I are coauthors, I use the first person when discussing my own patients, explaining herpes research, and providing medical recommendations.

Herpes Diseases and Your Health is dramatic, with romantic, mysterious, comic, and tragic scenes. Much of it is illustrated by case histories of patients; names and certain details have been altered to ensure anonymity. Parts of this drama may be painful for some readers, but my aim always is to provide the most up-to-date answers to your questions so that you can deal effectively with your medical problems. This book is not meant to be a self-treatment manual. Patients ill with herpesvirus infections need to consult their own physician for care. But I do want you to know as much about the herpes family as possible because "knowledge is power." Knowing what to look for and what to expect from herpesvirus infections is most of the battle. And there is good news. Many herpes diseases can be treated. I will tell you how.

If you have genital herpes, chapters 2 and 3 are written especially for you. If you have cold sores, chapter 4 offers helpful hints for handling them. Chickenpox and its complications are detailed in chapter 5. Shingles sufferers, chapter 6 is especially for you. If you are a student with mono and want to know if it's all right to date, be sure to read chapter 7. If you are pregnant and afraid that herpesviruses will damage your baby, pay close attention to chapters 3 and 8. Finally, if you are just plain curious about herpes diseases, read on, because the whole book was written for you.

H. H. B.

Acknowledgments / xi

Special thanks to Marian Wallfred for her assistance in preparing the manuscript; to William R. Hoffman and Candace Gulko for literary guidance; to L. Edward Kirk, Drs. Bonnie Bean, Patricia Ferrieri, Lawrence A. Lockman, Angeline Mastri, and John D. Nelson for reviewing certain portions of the manuscript; to Dr. Bud Tucker and other loyal physicians who referred patients to us for clinical trials; to Dr. Nancy Cole and Mary Albury-Noyes for medical art work; and to all the patients who participated in clinical investigations for the advancement of medical science.

HERPES DISEASES
and your health

Five in the Herpes Family

Herpes has become a household word, the result of saturation news coverage and the growing number of herpes sufferers. To some, herpes is a dirty word, *the* synonym for genital herpes and a symbol of sexual promiscuity. But herpes diseases take many forms besides genital sores, and most of them are not caught by genital contact. For example, chickenpox, which spreads through the air, is viewed as one of the rites of childhood. Doctors rarely tell us the name of the chickenpox virus or that it's similar to herpes. Nearly half of us will contract mononucleosis, which is caused by a herpesvirus that grows in the mouth, not on the genitals. Herpes diseases can be so mild that we have forgotten them by the time we reach adulthood. On the other hand, patients whose immunity is weakened by cancer or drugs may experience life-threatening herpesvirus infections that develop from trivial cold sores.

WHO SUFFERS FROM HERPES DISEASES?

Jeff and Jennifer, both in their thirties, struggled with feelings of guilt, anger, and despair because their sex lives were altered by venereal disease. They are victims of the genital herpes epidemic caused mostly by herpes simplex virus type 2, but occasionally by herpes simplex type 1.

Doug, a 29-year-old landscape architect, carries a stick of lip ice with him wherever he goes to minimize the irritation of recurrent cold sores. He is afflicted with herpes simplex type 1, the virus responsible for cold sores on the lips of an estimated 30 million Americans. In addition to the discomfort, Doug is now having trouble getting dates. But let me dispel one myth right away—you can't get genital herpes from a cold sore unless that cold sore touches your genitals.

At age 17 months, Carrie suddenly developed seizures that doctors could not control. She was referred to the University of Minnesota Hospitals, where neurosurgeons operated on her brain, expecting to find and remove a blood clot. Instead, they uncovered dead brain tissue containing herpes simplex virus type 1. Carrie had an infection of the brain termed herpes encephalitis.

When he was eight, Mike recovered from acute leukemia after receiving irradiation and powerful anticancer drugs. But 18 months later he was rushed from Florida to Minnesota in a desperate attempt to prevent him from breaking out in chickenpox. Chickenpox, usually a mild childhood illness, can be life threatening for children who have cancer. Chickenpox is caused by varicella-zoster virus, a bona fide member of the herpes family.

Lucille was 62 when the pain grew so intense that she ended her career as an antique dealer. Like many of the elderly, she endured the agony of shingles, a rash followed in some cases by persistent pain. Since her physicians could offer no solace and her pain was often unbearable, she contemplated suicide. Shingles, like chickenpox, is caused by varicella-zoster virus.

Kim, a vivacious 17-year-old cheerleader, missed a semester of high school because of a severe bout with mononucleosis. Mono, commonly known as the kissing disease, is caused by Epstein-Barr virus, the most recently discovered member of the herpes family. Kim tried to return to school too soon, as many mono victims do, and wound up back in bed.

Ted's kidneys failed when he was 40 and at the height of his executive career. The gift of a kidney from his older brother saved him. Ted's new kidney was functioning well and he was about to be discharged from the hospital when he developed a fever and pneumonia. He had been stricken by cytomegalovirus (CMV), the fifth and least-known member of the human herpesvirus family. CMV also causes birth defects and monolike illnesses.

In other words, herpes diseases affect almost everyone, from tiny tots to grandparents. I'll tell you more about the patients you've just met and introduce you to others in the following chapters. But first, let me provide some essential background about the peculiarities of the herpes family and how our bodies repel a viral attack.

WHAT DOES HERPES MEAN?

Herpes is derived from the Greek word *to creep*. In ancient days *herpes* meant a skin rash, no matter what the cause. Since many rashes enlarge and spread before they heal, the sores were thought to creep over the surface of our bodies. Now we know that most rashes are not herpes and that herpes is always more than skin deep. In this book *herpes* refers either to the herpes simplex viruses (type 1 and type 2) or to the illnesses they produce. *Herpes diseases* includes all ailments ascribed to the human herpes family. The term *herpesvirus* refers to any one of the five members of the human herpesvirus family:

- Herpes simplex virus type 1
- Herpes simplex virus type 2
- Varicella-zoster virus
- Epstein-Barr virus
- Cytomegalovirus

These closely related viruses look alike under the electron microscope and share important biological characteristics.

OFFENSE: THE VIRAL INVADERS

What exactly is a virus? Viruses are the smallest things we know of that may be called alive, yet they are the biggest killers in the universe. They are so small that they can cause diseases in bacteria. You have probably seen a red blood cell under the microscope. As many as 20,000 herpesviruses could fit inside that single cell! Unlike bacteria, viruses cannot function independently outside cells. They require the elaborate biochemical machinery of the host cell in order to multiply and cause disease.

First Attack

After attaching to and penetrating the host cell, the virus takes charge, turning the cell into a virus factory. Instead of going about the usual business of manufacturing its own materials, the host cell starts reproducing more viruses. In a way, our normal cells have been enslaved or reprogrammed.

A viral attack does not automatically spell victory for the invaders. Three factors are always involved: the amount of virus transmitted (called the inoculum), the capacity of the viral strain to produce disease (called virulence), and the individual's ability to fight off the attack (the immune response).

Latency and Recurrence

All herpesviruses possess a unique behavioral trait that allows them to survive, whereas other viruses, such as polio and rubella, are easily eradicated. Latency, or the ability to hibernate following the primary infection, makes herpesviruses particularly difficult to eliminate.

Where does the virus hide? Epstein-Barr virus establishes latency inside specialized white blood cells called B-lymphocytes. CMV hides so well that no scientist has yet discovered its resting place. Both herpes simplex and varicella-zoster viruses travel along the nerve pathways until they reach the ganglia, collections of nerve cell bodies located along

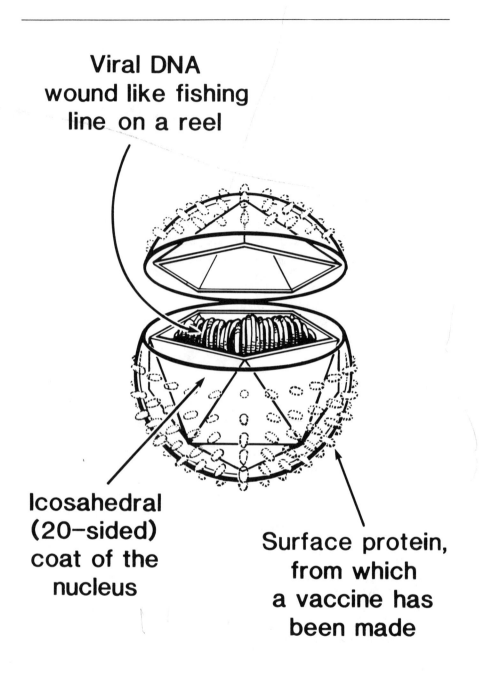

Viral DNA wound like fishing line on a reel

Icosahedral (20–sided) coat of the nucleus

Surface protein, from which a vaccine has been made

A portrait of the herpesvirus. All five members of the human herpes family look alike.

the spine and near the base of the brain. The viral particles (called virions) climb inside cell bodies and remain there dormant or sleeping. While in hiding the viruses produce no symptoms and are probably not contagious. When a sudden stimulus awakens the virions, they multiply, travel back along nerve pathways, and once again cause symptoms. Now the individual is contagious.

Any herpesvirus can resurface later in life following a period of latency. We know that this will occur if the immune system has been weakened, for example, in the case of the transplant patient. We can't always predict whether the virus will reemerge in normal patients, though we do recognize some stimuli that trigger recurrences: stress, sunshine, fatigue, menses, fever, masturbation.

THE IMMUNE DEFENSE

Our major line of defense is the body's immune system, consisting of complex armies and navies of antibodies and white blood cells. The immune system recognizes foreign invaders—be they wood slivers, bacteria, or viruses—and musters an effective biological arsenal in its defense.

Without the vast array of cells and molecules in the immune system, we could not survive infancy. Even the most inoffensive bacteria would wreak havoc in our bodies, eventually causing death. We see this in children born with Severe Combined Immune Deficiency who usually die from infection within a few months after losing the temporary immunity passed on from their mothers at birth.

The immune defense is one of nature's marvelous creations. More than one trillion white blood cells float through the bloodstream on constant alert for any foreign element. Our body reacts to the viral offense by unleashing an armada of white blood cells. Certain white blood cells (polys) engulf and eat invading viruses. Others (macrophages) alter the viruses in such a way that yet another type of white cell (the lymphocyte) recognizes the virus material as foreign and makes antibodies to attack it. The antibody molecule is shaped to fit over the virus, preventing the invader from parasitizing our cells. Once virus has been spotted and attacked by the immune defense, specialized lymphocytes are taught to memorize distinctive parts of the virus called antigens. This immune memory stays with us the rest of our lives. When we experience a second attack by the same virus, our immune system remembers the first encounter and reacts more swiftly. This is why recurrent episodes of herpetic infections usually are shorter and milder than the first.

We know that our immune system provides vital protection against herpesvirus infections, because the herpes family is the most common cause of serious infections in patients whose immunity is deliberately damaged. Patients in need of a new kidney are given drugs right before transplantation to prevent their immune system from recognizing the donated organ as foreign and rejecting it. They are then "immunosuppressed." We can predict, almost like clockwork, when kidney transplant patients will erupt with herpesvirus infections. Herpes simplex comes within days after transplantation, CMV within weeks, and varicella-zoster within months. The immune defense, once strong and able to keep the latent viruses at bay, has been weakened, and the viral offense wins the day.

Now that I've introduced the human herpesvirus family and the concept of the viral offense versus the immune defense, let's consider herpes diseases in more detail. In the following chapters I'll tell you when to suspect that you have a herpesvirus infection, where to go for help, what to do for yourself, and what progress medical science is making toward prevention, treatment, and a cure. This knowledge will help you avoid getting sick. If you're already afflicted, complete information can give you power over your disease, easing your road to recovery.

Let's begin with genital herpes. How we catch genital herpes can be puzzling, because herpes' source is not always obvious. If you enjoy a good mystery story, read on. The next chapter will whet your detective instincts by tracing the sometimes puzzling path of herpes simplex.

Genital Herpes:
How Do We Catch It?

Mothers refuse to launder their infected children's linens. Women won't try on department store lipstick. Sales of disinfectants are sky-rocketing. Herpes is cited as proof of infidelity. Marriages are dissolving. Noninfected individuals shun all contact with previously infected people—even children who had neonatal herpes years ago. Exclusive dating services are forming, some for members who have herpes, and some for those who don't. We have witnessed all these trends in our society since *herpes* became a household word. They result from blatant misconceptions about how the virus is spread. Some myths are even based on reports in medical journals. For example . . .

THE HOT TUB DEBATE HEATS UP

Browsing through their morning newspapers on December 9, 1983, millions of Americans saw alarming headlines on possible nonvenereal herpes transmission in public areas. The press was reporting on an article in that week's issue of the *Journal of the American Medical Association* titled "Survival of Herpes Simplex Virus in Water Specimens Collected from Hot Tubs in Spa Facilities and on Plastic Surfaces."

The authors of the article were scientists at the National Institutes of Health (NIH) in Bethesda, Maryland, who launched their investigation into herpes survival following reports of possible transmission of herpes simplex infections at commercial spas in the Washington, D.C., area. A number of health spa patrons had complained of contracting herpes following use of the facilities.

The public health nature of the study obviously would spark widespread interest, even panic, among uninfected men and women who use public showers; it also rekindled a debate among virologists and other scientists who did not totally accept the NIH findings. Was the public unnecessarily panicked by these stories? If so, who was responsible: the press or the scientists who conducted the study? Let's examine the situation.

The government researchers, headed by Dr. Lata S. Nerurkar, said that herpes did not survive in samples of spa water because the water contained high levels of chlorine and bromine which killed the micro-organisms. However, the study did prove that a *laboratory strain* of herpes simplex type 2 (the type most often responsible for genital herpes) could survive up to four and one-half hours on moist plastic surfaces similar to locker room benches. The researchers concluded: "The persistence of viruses on plastic suggests that these surfaces might provide a route for nonvenereal spread of HSV (herpes simplex virus)."

What's wrong with that conclusion? First, laboratory strains are not the same as human strains. A laboratory strain might survive for a longer period outside the body because this form of virus is grown outside the body in flasks of tissue cultures. Second, it is highly unlikely that herpes can penetrate normal skin. Breaks in the skin tissue or trauma to the mucous membrane surface of the mouth or genitals are probably required to permit virus to enter our body. Third, the NIH scientists did not perform the ultimate experiment: to have a volunteer (and I believe it would be very hard to find such a subject) sit on the herpes-infected plastic bench and actually acquire the virus from the surface.

Drs. John M. Douglas and Lawrence Corey, genital herpes researchers at the University of Washington, Seattle, pointed out these problems in an editorial accompanying the research report. Unfortunately, the headlines and many of the news stories devoted scant attention to the editorial, nearly condemning spas as out of bounds for clean-living citizens. Douglas and Corey wrote:

> While Nerurkar and others have demonstrated that HSV can survive on wet cloth or plastic for several hours . . . these observations do not provide proof that fomites [objects capable of harboring infectious organisms] play a role in the transmission of genital herpes. . . . Even if virus can persist in the environment, for transmission to occur, a series of logistic hurdles must be crossed: the inoculation of a flat surface from a vulvar or penile lesion, the subsequent contact with the infectious secretion by another person, and the deposition of this infectious material on an epidermal [skin] or mucosal surface followed by enough of a mechanical "irritation" to facilitate infection. Such a sequence of events makes transmission by fomites unlikely.

In summary, both the authors of the article *and* the press were responsible for the "spa panic." The authors overextended their conclusions and the press largely ignored Douglas and Corey's sensible caveats concerning direct application of laboratory results to the actual spa setting.

A more comprehensive set of experiments concerning survival of herpes on artificial surfaces was carried out by Drs. Trudy Larson and Yvonne Bryson. These scientists from the University of California at Los Angeles showed that herpes could survive on a toilet seat for up to one and one-half hours after being placed on the surface. Their experiment involved strains of virus taken directly from patients. Samples of virus were collected from 10 patients, then rubbed on a ceramic toilet seat. Also, one patient with active herpes sat on the toilet seat. Although herpes simplex was recovered, the clinching experiment again was not done: a healthy human volunteer was not exposed to the virus to learn if herpes actually could be caught from a toilet seat.

A group of scientists from the University of Minnesota and the Minneapolis Veterans Administration Hospital, headed by Dr. Bonnie Bean, conducted similar studies using influenza virus. They showed that influenza, too, survives on inanimate surfaces — not for hours, but for days! In theoretically calculating the amount of influenza necessary to be transmitted from an artificial surface to the hands, and thence to the nose or mouth in order to infect, they determined you would have to touch the virus-containing surface within 15 minutes of its initial contamination. Otherwise, too little virus was present to transmit flu.

Herpes simplex survives in the environment for a shorter period than influenza does. Although the theoretical possibility exists that if a large amount of herpes was deposited on a plastic bench, persons might become infected if their genitals touched the bench shortly thereafter, I believe that spas and public toilet seats are safe. The bottom line on nonvenereal transmission of genital herpes: improbable but remotely possible. Yet the fear of transmission to innocent people persists, even affecting decisions of who can attend school.

"HERPES HYSTERIA" VICTIMIZES A FOUR-YEAR-OLD

A four-year-old girl from Emporia, Kansas, handicapped at birth with neonatal herpes, was one of many victims of "herpes hysteria" emanating from widespread misunderstanding of transmission. In 1983, administrators of the school district's Severely and Multiply Handicapped program attempted to exclude the child from enrollment for fear she would infect her classmates. Only after the federal Centers for

Disease Control (CDC) and state health officials intervened, providing scientific proof that her class was not at risk, did the school board relent and allow the little girl into class. The community outcry at the decision, which news reports described as a "prevailing panic," revealed the deep-seeded myths about herpes diseases.

In the aftermath of the school board's decision, Dr. Mary Guinan, the CDC researcher who submitted data to the Emporia school board, reportedly was besieged with phone calls from women who were worried about becoming infected, conceiving, and delivering a damaged infant. She was quoted as saying that many more physicians are likely to be confronted with similar situations in the future because of false notions of transmission.

TRANSMISSION OF HERPES—FOUR EXAMPLES

Tracking the spread of genital herpes requires good medical detective work, termed epidemiology, backed by a well-equipped virology laboratory. To involve you in the spirit of scientific inquiry and discovery, here are four mysterious cases from my personal experience, followed by clues that lead to the proper diagnosis.

An Athlete's Story of Genital Herpes

In the spring of 1982, during a peak period of local media coverage of the genital herpes story, including reports that a new antiviral drug was being studied at the University of Minnesota, many young people with genital sores referred themselves to our special research group. They came to us seeking treatment with a medication still in the experimental stage.

The Case: One of the more unusual cases was Paul, a member of the University football team, who had a typical herpes simplex type 2 illness: fever, lesions on the shaft of his penis, swollen lymph glands, and a generalized achiness. When I advised Paul that he indeed had genital herpes, he could not understand how he contracted the disease. "I'm certain I don't have herpes because I've read that the rash starts six days after exposure," he said. "The last time I had sexual relations was 30 days ago, and this rash just developed yesterday."

The Mystery: If Paul's last sexual encounter was a month before the onset of fever, blisters, and soreness, could he really have genital herpes? If so, why did it take so long for symptoms to surface?

Clue: Genital lesions usually start within a week of exposure, according to the most complete study by researchers at the University of Washington in Seattle. However, the incubation period of genital herpes may be as long as a month, and the first episode sometimes can be so mild that the patient is unaware of a problem. About 30 percent of the patients do not recognize their primary attack. Such unrecognized attacks are termed "asymptomatic."

Solution: We drew some blood from Paul's arm and brought the sample to our virus laboratory for testing. The laboratory technologist looked for specific antibodies — protein molecules made when the immune system encounters a virus. Since these antibodies don't appear until several weeks after the first infection, their presence would prove this was not Paul's first encounter with herpes. The test found antibody against herpes. Paul had, indeed, suffered an earlier episode of genital herpes, albeit so mild he didn't recognize it.

The Mystery: From whom did Paul acquire genital herpes and what triggered his symptomatic episode after a first asymptomatic one?

Clue: We have witnessed a definite link between emotional stress and the recurrence of genital herpes.

Solution: Paul was under a great deal of pressure when he came to see us. In addition to spring workouts for varsity football, he was preparing for exam week *and* attempting to find a summer job in order to pay for next year's tuition. I counseled Paul about the social consequences of genital herpes and encouraged him to discuss the situation with Chris, his sexual partner of a month ago. I suspected she was unaware that she harbored the virus. If Chris was the carrier, she might have recurrences and could infect others. When Paul later talked with Chris, she remembered that she had pain during urination in the past — a common symptom of herpes in women — but ignored it.

Comment: The epidemic of venereal herpes has recast many physicians as social psychologists. In addition to treating illness, they must offer emotional reassurance to their patients. To some, this metamorphosis from the traditional role of physical healer to mental health counselor is uncomfortable; medical schools tend to focus on physiology rather than psychology. But to deal properly with a rampant viral epidemic intimately linked to sexual mores one must understand the social dynamics of the time.

Paul returned for a checkup about a week later. The blisters on his penis were gone, and he reported feeling fit again. But he became very depressed when I explained that the sores were likely to recur. He was mad at Chris for giving him herpes; he said he was embarrassed to discuss herpes with his friends. This young man, like others who are victims of the herpedemic, needed an outlet for his pent-up rage. For some victims, unraveling the mystery, discovering what the infection is and where it came from, provides relief. For others, the solution is an emotional powderkeg, charged with hostility, distrust, and blame directed at the sex partner who infected them.

Paul and I talked for nearly an hour about social diseases, personal hygiene, and other possible ways of preventing another herpes outbreak. By the end of the appointment, Paul's need for knowledge seemed satisfied, but his emotions remained in turmoil. I suggested that he contact the University's Student Health Service where the mental health group offered a special "talk session" just for herpes sufferers.

Genital Herpes from a Kiss?

The front page of a national scandal sheet screams: "MOVIE ACTRESS REFUSES TO KISS ON THE SET—FEARS GENITAL HERPES." At first glance the headline seems ridiculous. Since the movie production was not X-rated, we assume the starlet was afraid to kiss an actor on the mouth. She couldn't catch genital herpes by kissing someone's lips, or could she? The following story about a patient of mine helps answer this question.

The Case: A faculty colleague of mine, whom I'll call Bill, came to me with the following story: except for a childhood bout with chickenpox, he never had problems with herpesviruses until now. One evening, while he attended a cocktail party, the partygoers became very expressive. As he was saying goodnight to the hostess, she gave him a juicy and probing kiss on the mouth. As they separated, Bill noticed a large cold sore on the woman's lower lip. He thought no more of it.

Seven days later, Bill became acutely ill with oral herpes—blisters on his lip and ulcers in his mouth and on his gums. He had a fever and was so sick he couldn't work for two days, but totally recovered within a week.

Feeling perfectly well again, he became sexually involved with a friend named Mary. A week later she called him to complain: "Bill, I think I got genital herpes. I know I've got genital herpes, and I'm sure I caught it from you." Bill disputed her claim, but she persisted in her contention. Her gynecologist cultured the lesions in her vagina, and the lab report came back "herpes simplex type 1 isolated."

The Mystery: Bill had no signs of genital herpes, yet the gynecologist confirmed that Mary did. Could she have caught it from Bill? In other words, can a person with oral herpes give a sex partner genital herpes?

Clue: The viruses responsible for oral herpes and genital herpes are very similar. Type 1 herpes generally causes cold sores and eye infections, type 2 genital herpes. But with changing sexual practices, these distinctions are not clear-cut. Oral herpes can be due to the type 2 virus, and genital herpes to type 1.

Solution: During my interview with Bill, he acknowledged that he and Mary had engaged in oral-genital sex. I asked if both partners or just one performed oral sex. Unless Bill had performed cunnilingus (oral contact with Mary's genitals), she could not have caught genital herpes from Bill's mouth. Bill said that he had indeed performed cunnilingus. Therefore, I reasoned that he infected her genital tract with virus-containing oral secretions which later resulted in painful vaginal blisters.

To confirm the diagnosis, I asked Bill to notify me if he developed cold sores on his lips or even a minor irritation of his gums. Within a few weeks, he called to report a tingling in his gums that was aggravated by brushing his teeth. We swabbed Bill's mouth and sent the culture specimen to our lab. The lab confirmed that he had herpes simplex type 1.

Comment: Herpes type 1 can cause genital infections similar to herpes type 2. It is possible to be completely asymptomatic during a recurrent episode of oral herpes. Bill transmitted his herpes strain to Mary's genitals even though he had no recognizable signs or symptoms of oral herpes at that time.

Bill's story proves the movie actress's fears were not totally unfounded. She could catch oral herpes by kissing a person with active herpes. During her first attack of oral herpes, she could spread the virus by touching her mouth and then her own genitals. Or, if she performed oral-genital sex while her mouth sores were active, she could give a sex partner genital herpes.

Herpes in the Newborn

Doctors and nurses who care for pregnant women are constantly on the alert for herpes infections. We estimate the incidence of herpes in the newborn (neonatal herpes) to be one in 7,500 live births, or approximately 500 babies in the United States every year. Though rare, the condition is serious: about half of all cases are fatal unless treated with antiviral drugs.

The Case: Mrs. Linda Whitmore, age 24, attended our Childbearing and Childrearing Clinic for regular classes and examinations during her pregnancy. She reported no history of genital herpes, and her physical exam revealed no hint of herpes. About a week before delivery, she felt vaguely uncomfortable (doctors refer to this as malaise). The discomfort left her as subtly as it had come. Mrs. Whitmore delivered eight-pound Jonathan without complications. The young mother chose to breast-feed him beginning early the next day. Upon bringing Jonathan to his mother for his initial feeding, an alert nurse heard something disturbing—the baby had an unusually high-pitched cry. She notified the pediatrician on call, who observed some abnormal reflexes when he examined the infant. The physician deduced incipient encephalitis and immediately placed Jonathan in the intensive care unit for careful monitoring. The working medical diagnosis was neonatal herpes; this form of herpes infection often involves the brain.

The Mystery: Herpes in the mother's genital tract can invade the baby's tiny body during birth. Viral particles shed from the mother can also infect the baby during cuddling or feeding after birth. But Mrs. Whitmore reported no history of herpes and showed no signs of genital blisters. What happened?

Clue: Many of the women whose babies develop neonatal herpes lack visible lesions. This is the case at least 50 percent of the time. Mrs. Whitmore's malaise preceding delivery may have been a herpes attack. To confirm our suspicions that the mother had recurrent genital herpes, we touched her vagina and cervix with cotton-tipped swabs and sent them to the virus laboratory for culture.

Clue: Two days after birth, Jonathan developed mouth sores— another sign of a herpes infection. We sent swabs from the baby's mouth to our lab for viral cultures.

Solution: Cultures taken from the mother and baby were positive for herpes simplex type 2. To try to protect Jonathan from permanent brain damage, we immediately started him on an intravenous infusion with the antiviral drug vidarabine. Within a few days his lesions were gone, and two weeks later he was discharged from the hospital in normal condition. At age two, Jonathan is perfectly normal in physical growth and mental development, but he suffers occasional cold sores on the lip.

The Mystery: Mrs. Whitmore could not account for the source of her herpes infection. An antibody test of the father proved negative.

Clue: Genital herpes can recur for many, many years. The later the recurrence, the more likely it will be mild or even asymptomatic.

Solution: We requestioned Mrs. Whitmore about her medical history after establishing the diagnosis of neonatal herpes. She mentioned suffering from genital sores after a relationship a few years before her marriage. We'll never know for sure, but we suspect that bout was genital herpes. She had no obvious recurrences for many years, but something apparently triggered the onset of a subtle recurrent infection late in pregnancy.

Comment: Herpes in the newborn is rare, but potentially dangerous. Not appreciating this, Mrs. Whitmore concealed an important part of her medical history from us. If you're pregnant, be sure to tell your doctor if you or your sex partner ever had any sores or discomfort that you think might have been genital herpes. Your doctor will be alert for evidence of herpes in you or your baby and will handle the situation appropriately. (More on this in chapter 3.)

Robert and the Finger

Many doctors and nurses believe they have a special immunity that protects them from their patients' diseases. Although not true, this notion helps ensure good patient care. Imagine doctors refusing to examine you because they don't want your cold! Sometimes, however, medical personnel become a little careless and then . . .

The Case: Robert was an M.D. in his final year of pediatric residency at the "U." As Robert's academic adviser, I helped guide his clinical and research work. Following one of our regular meetings to discuss a complicated case, Robert asked me for some advice about his own medical problem.

Robert explained: "My wife, Cammy, lately refuses to kiss me because I have cold sores on my lip. I never had oral herpes before, and I think I got it from a two-year-old patient. When I explained to Cammy that the oral herpes simplex virus is similar to but different from the genital version, she became very upset and accused me of having an affair. I have been faithful to her, but how can I prove that I don't have VD?"

Robert often examines children who suffer from herpes infections of the mouth. He has even hospitalized patients because their pain was so intense that they refused to take liquids. In the hospital, patients receive intravenous fluids until the mouth sores heal, usually within a week. Two weeks before we talked, Robert was examining a child with a particularly bad case of mouth sores. In the course of the examination, he tore the plastic glove covering his right hand. The gloves provided a measure of safety and comfort for Robert. First, they protected him (and the next patient he examined) from many transmittable diseases. Second, because he was a chronic nail biter, the tight-fitting gloves offered a soothing sensation over his rough and sometimes bleeding cuticles.

The Mystery: How could the virus from the child penetrate Robert's skin?

Clue: Herpes can be transmitted from an open sore to the fingers. Health care personnel dealing with patients with active cases of herpes run the risk of contracting the disease in this way. A simple cut or scratch can serve as an entry point for the virus. On examination, Robert had what resembled a small healing abscess on his right index finger beside the nail.

Solution: Robert's glove was torn, and there was a break in the skin of his index finger. Viral particles from the child's mouth seeped into Robert's finger through the cut cuticle. The abscesslike sore on his index finger is typical of a herpes infection called herpetic whitlow. Robert had transferred herpes from his finger to his mouth by biting his nails shortly after examining the patient. After a week's incubation period, he developed herpes sores simultaneously in his mouth and on his finger. Our laboratory cultured herpes simplex type 1 from Robert's finger. Robert had oral herpes and herpetic whitlow—not genital herpes.

Comment: Cold sores are contagious. Any minor abrasion such as a cut around the cuticle allows the virus to enter the body. Even one viral particle may cause a problem because it can reproduce until there is a sufficient amount of virus in the body to cause acute illness. After tearing his glove in the course of the examination, Robert still could have protected himself by washing his hands. This, he confessed to me, he had neglected to do. Herpetic whitlow is primarily a nuisance, but it can lead to more serious infections if, for example, you touch your eye with an infected finger. If you touch the genitals of a person who has never had herpes, genital herpes could result. Whitlows usually last two to six weeks and recur less frequently than oral or genital herpes.

Robert and Cammy worked through their marital crisis, eventually laughing about the unusual way Robert caught oral herpes: "We never imagined a sick patient, nail-biting, and a torn glove would make us stop kissing!"

Seriously, active cold sores of the lip and mouth put your spouse at risk. I do not recommend mouth-to-mouth contact until your herpes lip and mouth sores have completely healed.

EPIDEMIOLOGY: HOW HERPES IS "CAUGHT"

Herpes spreads by human-to-human contact—direct touching of the mucous membranes of the lips, eyes, or genitals. You're most likely to catch genital herpes during sexual contact with someone who has active herpes sores. Herpes can be transmitted by any type of genital contact with the viral carrier. You may become infected during sexual intercourse, oral-genital sex, anal intercourse, and even the skin-to-skin rubbing of your genitalia.

Incorrect self-diagnosis has contributed to the continuing spread of genital herpes. You may mistake malaise for a touch of the flu, rather than herpes simplex. The initial episode of genital herpes may be so mild that you fail to recognize any symptoms. You are then likely to pass on the virus to someone else, unintentionally of course.

As I've just said, you may shed the virus into your oral or genital secretions without having any sores or symptoms. This presents a dilemma for all individuals including those involved in long-term monogamous relationships. Even if you are very careful and abstain from sex when your herpes is active, your partner may still become infected. However, recent scientific evidence suggests that you are much more likely to pass herpes to a sex partner when you have fresh herpes sores and that you become *less* contagious as the sores heal. Since sores usually heal more quickly during recurrences, you tend to become less contagious as time goes on.

The risk of genital herpes, except in instances of child abuse, doesn't start until an individual becomes sexually active. Babies may acquire herpes from their mothers. In these unusual cases, babies most often are infected during birth from virus in maternal genital secretions.

Once we have herpes, the virus never totally leaves our bodies. The primary episode is usually the worst, but recurrent attacks can be quite painful and irritating. Subsequent attacks are almost always reactivations of our own virus. The triggering mechanism may be stress, poor nutrition, a suppressed immune system, or other factors still unknown. Seventy-five percent of patients with genital herpes have recurrences about every three months.

THE HERPEDEMIC

Epidemiologists, for the most part, go about their work quietly, tracking disease outbreaks in the field, analyzing data, and looking for trends. The fruits of their labor—dissemination of information to the general public—will, they hope, safeguard the unprotected. Once in a while they become the focus of media attention, such as during the Philadelphia outbreak of Legionnaires' Disease in 1976. The United States Public Health Service mobilized a cadre of epidemiologists to find the cause and prevent further outbreaks of the mysterious and often lethal illness. Genital herpes does not possess the life-threatening characteristics of the *Legionella* bacterium, but its rapid spread certainly has posed a public health threat to some and a chronic medical problem to many others.

Epidemiologists tracing the spread of genital herpes have decided that there is indeed a national epidemic. The official declaration came on March 26, 1982, when the Atlanta-based CDC announced in the publication *Morbidity and Mortality Weekly Report* that the virus outbreak had reached "epidemic" proportions. Though the announcement was only seven paragraphs long, its impact on the medical community was profound. It read, in part:

> *CDC has analyzed data on genital herpes infection. . . . This analysis supports the widely held contention that an epidemic of genital herpes infection occurred in the United States from 1966 to 1979 — the most recent year[s] for which data are available.*
>
> *The estimated number and rate of consultations with physicians for genital herpes infection both increased markedly from 1966 to 1979. The number of consultations for genital herpes infection increased from 29,560 in 1966 to 260,890 in 1979. The rate at which patients consulted fee-for-service office-based physicians for* **genital herpes infection increased almost 9-fold** *[emphasis added] from 3.4 per 100,000 consultations in 1966 to 29.2 per 100,000 in 1979.*

The CDC observed that social, demographic, and behavioral changes during the 1970s placed an increased proportion of the population at risk for sexually transmitted diseases.

An epidemic means rapid spread of a disease among many individuals in the same community. In other words, the incidence of the disease is on the rise. The accompanying graph, adapted from the latest available CDC statistics, illustrates that there truly is an epidemic of genital herpes in the United States. Notice the sharp upward trend for genital herpes, compared with the slopes for gonorrhea and syphilis. Efforts to control gonorrhea were intensified in 1973 and may be responsible for slowing its increase. Cases of syphilis and gonorrhea were tabulated from a different data base than genital herpes, because gonorrhea and syphilis are reportable communicable diseases in the United

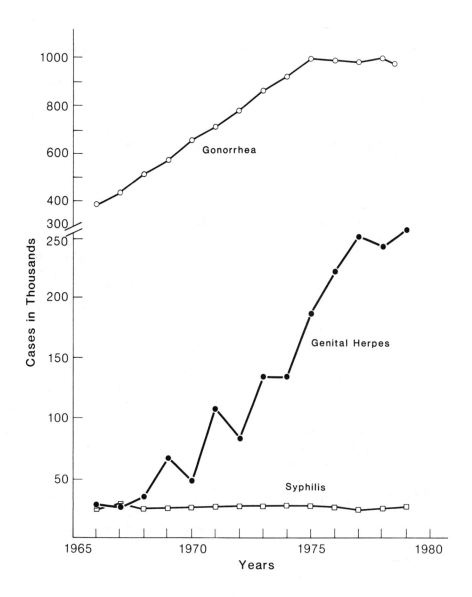

Cases of venereal disease in the United States between 1966 and 1979. Adapted from statistics provided by the Centers for Disease Control.

States, whereas herpes is not. Estimated numbers of genital herpes cases were based on reports from physicians in private practice rather than on public health records. Since patients cared for in public health facilities, outpatient clinics, and hospital emergency rooms were not included in the genital herpes survey, the absolute number of genital herpes cases probably far exceeds the number shown on the graph.

The latest CDC report estimates 600,000 new cases of genital herpes per year. Although awareness and new treatment probably will stem the tidal wave, the herpedemic will remain with us for some time. What factors led to the herpedemic? Why did the problem become acute in the late 1970s, rather than the 1960s or before?

Most virus experts and epidemiologists believe the rampant spread of genital herpes originated in the so-called sexual revolution of the 1960s. Two major events of that decade changed sexual practices in the United States. The development of an effective birth control pill *and* liberalized abortion laws unquestionably allowed more sexual freedom. That freedom permitted more sexual partners. And with more sexual partners, the likelihood of venereal disease was enhanced.

The pill was approved by the federal Food and Drug Administration in May 1960, but it was several years before the contraceptive gained widespread use. Abortion was legalized by the U.S. Supreme Court in 1973 after a number of states had passed liberalized laws governing abortion, beginning with Colorado in 1967. Genital herpes certainly existed at that time, but not until the mid-1960s did the virus become prevalent in the population. More cases of syphilis and gonorrhea were also observed during the 1970s, but the impact of their increase was less frightening than that of genital herpes because those bacterial diseases respond to antibiotics.

Several other factors helped fuel the epidemic. First, children born during the baby boom of the post-World War II era became sexually active adults in the late sixties and early seventies. Put bluntly, more people in the United States were having sex than at any time before, many with a variety of partners.

Changes were taking place in the institutions of marriage and family during the 1960s and 1970s. Young people tended to delay their first marriages during the two decades—the median age at wedlock increased from 22.5 to 23.4 for men and from 20.4 to 21.6 for women between 1965 and 1980. Divorce rates increased dramatically during the period as the proportion of divorced people climbed from 3 to 7 percent.

Another reason for the epidemic may have something to do with our reluctance to seek medical help, even when we're sick. Many people with genital herpes, as well as other forms of VD, fail to seek prompt medical assistance. In a 10-month study of callers to a national VD Hotline, researchers learned that only 48.1 percent of the callers accepted and followed through on a referral to a medical facility. More than half were not sure they would go to a doctor, delayed the visit, or ignored the referral suggestion altogether. Of course, we suspect some of those callers eventually did seek aid. But certainly some did not, and they contributed to the herpedemic. (Of the callers, 38 percent were believed to have genital herpes, 33 percent gonorrhea, 13 percent syphilis, and the remaining 16 percent had miscellaneous and less com- common types of VD.) In questioning by VD Hotline counselors, the callers who refused the referral said they did so out of fear of humiliation or anxiety over treatment.

Incorrect diagnosis has also contributed to the new epidemic. Not recognizing the illness as herpes leads some to continue to be sexually active during times when their herpes is infectious. In some cases, patients make erroneous self-diagnoses. At times doctors themselves fail to correctly identify genital herpes. To stem the herpedemic, I urge you not to try to diagnose yourself. See your own medical doctor. If you are uncomfortable with your doctor's diagnosis and management, seek a second opinion. Doctors must do their part by attending Continuing Medical Education programs to ensure that genital herpes and other "new" infectious diseases are recognized and dealt with promptly.

A sustaining factor in the herpedemic is the frequency of unrecog- nized recurrences. Recurrent genital herpes may be so mild that you don't realize you're sick, and inadvertently infect a sexual partner.

Genital herpes is so prevalent in our society that not every victim has to be promiscuous to become infected. Doctors, counselors, and even Ann Landers have received letter after letter from virgins catching herpes after first encounters, and from monogamous people infected by their spouses.

CATCHING HERPES: THE TOP 20 QUESTIONS

A diagnosis of genital herpes naturally provokes questions—often intimate ones. Most queries focus on the mode of transmission, possible complications, and new forms of treatment. Discussion of sexual prac- tices can be awkward, even for a physician. But, in my opinion, patients deserve frankness and facts.

Q. How am I most likely to catch genital herpes?

A. You acquire genital herpes from a sex partner who has an active case of herpes. The virus enters your body through mucous membranes—the soft tissues around your genital area. Genital herpes almost always results from genital-to-genital contact. Sometimes, as happened in Bill's case, oral-genital contact may transmit disease.

Q. Are there any exceptions?

A. We believe that genital herpes is caught only by direct person-to-person contact. The medical literature chronicles several situations in which herpes infection occurred without direct contact. All involved infants in a hospital setting. The case with the firmest documentation occurred in 1976 in a newborn nursery at the Cincinnati Children's Hospital Medical Center. Presumably, a caregiver or visitor transmitted the virus from one child, who was infected with herpes simplex type 1, to a second, infection-free baby. The babies never touched each other. Transmission of herpes in the nursery is unique because infants' immune systems are not fully developed, making them more susceptible to infections than adults are.

Q. Is it true that two viruses can cause genital herpes?

A. Yes. There are two types of herpes simplex. Herpes type 1 usually causes oral herpes and type 2, genital herpes. However, Bill's story indicated that genital herpes can be caught by having oral-genital sex with someone who has herpes simplex type 1 in his or her mouth. Both herpes type 1 and type 2 can cause genital herpes. Conversely, both types can cause oral herpes.

Q. Does my sex partner always know if he or she is infected?

A. No. Although we believe that genital herpes is most contagious during symptomatic periods, the disease can also spread when symptoms are mild or absent. In the story about the college athlete, Paul apparently was infected by an asymptomatic sexual partner.

Q. Will I automatically catch herpes by having intercourse with an infected sex partner?

A. No. Contracting herpes depends on several factors: the stage of infection in your partner, which determines the amount of virus transmitted; the presence of breaks in your skin or mucous membranes that permit virus to enter your body; and whether or not you are immune to herpes due to previous infection.

Q. Do condoms protect me from contracting and spreading herpes?

A. The shield offers some safety as long as it is not torn. However, genital herpes has been spread even when condoms were used.

Condoms will only protect the area that is covered. Your thighs and buttocks may become infected if enough virus contaminates cuts or abrasions on the unprotected skin surface.

Q. Can I catch herpes from the toilet seat?

A. Only if you get on before the last person got off. Although herpes can survive on toilet seats, transmission to human beings requires person-to-person contact. Most herpes experts do not believe that herpes can be caught from toilet seats, spa benches, lipstick, towels, washcloths, furniture, bathroom glasses, or any other nonhuman source. Nevertheless, for good personal hygiene, I do not recommend sharing drinking glasses or towels.

Q. Can I catch herpes from myself?

A. Yes. In a way, recurrence is the same as catching the virus from yourself. Something in your body reactivates the viral attack. You can also spread the virus from one part of your body to another. This process, called autoinoculation, was evident in the story of Robert, who gave himself cold sores by biting a newly infected finger. You are much more likely to infect other parts of your body, especially your mouth, eyes, or fingers, during your first episode of genital herpes because your immune system has not yet learned to recognize the virus and destroy it quickly.

Q. What risk do I run of having a recurrence of genital herpes?

A. Recurrences approximately every three months are reported in 80 percent of patients with genital herpes due to herpes type 2. In genital herpes due to type 1 virus, you have a 50 percent chance of recurrences, with an average frequency of one per year. Although firm scientific evidence is lacking, physicians and patients report that recurrences become less frequent and less severe over time.

Q. Where does genital herpes hide between recurrences?

A. The virus creeps along the nerve pathways to the base of the spine. It hibernates in collections of nerve cell bodies called ganglia until an impulse awakens the sleeping virus and sends it back along the nerve pathways to the genital area.

Q. Is herpes forever?

A. Yes and no. The virus remains in your body for the rest of your life, but that does not mean you will experience recurrent episodes year after year. As I said before, some people never have a recurrence of genital herpes, and recurrent episodes tend to become milder.

Q. Can I be infected with herpes a second time from another sex partner?

A. Yes. If you've been infected with type 1, you can still acquire type 2. Being immune to type 1 provides some measure of protection, but you could still catch type 2 virus, if you have sex with someone who is heavily infected. To complicate the situation further, many strains of herpes simplex exist. Even when you've been infected with and developed immunity to strain A, you may not be 100 percent immune to strain B.

Q. I work in a clinic with herpes patients. How can I protect myself?

A. Spread of herpesviruses requires close person-to-person contact. You never catch herpes by being in the same room or the same clinic with a patient. If you examine actual lesions of patients, you should wear gloves because herpes can, as it did in Robert's case, enter your body through a cut on the finger. The most important thing you can do to protect yourself and other patients from all viruses, not only herpes, is to wash your hands thoroughly after each examination.

Q. Am I at greater risk of catching herpes because I use birth control pills?

A. If your partner has active genital herpes and does not use a condom because you are on birth control pills, you are more likely to become infected. I don't recommend sex when *either* partner has active genital herpes in any case. The pill itself contains steroid hormones. These have a suppressive effect on our immune system. Therefore, birth control pills theoretically could enhance our susceptibility to genital herpes. No scientific studies have been published to support or refute this.

Q. Are homosexuals more susceptible than heterosexuals to herpes infections?

A. No. Although the incidence of all venereal diseases is higher in the homosexual population, we do not believe this group is intrinsically more susceptible to herpesviruses. Their risk of acquiring genital herpes is greater than that of the general population because they average more sex partners. In addition, anal herpes poses a problem for male homosexuals who practice rectal intercourse.

Q. Does genital herpes make me more vulnerable to other forms of venereal disease?

A. No. Herpes does not lead directly to syphilis and gonorrhea. However, your risk of multiple VD infections increases with increasing numbers of sex partners.

Q. I have herpes. How can I help stem the herpes epidemic?

A. In other words, how can you keep your herpes to yourself? If you have genital herpes, avoid sexual contact from the time you recognize the first symptoms until the sores are completely healed and the skin or mucous membranes return to normal appearance.

Q. How do babies contract herpes?

A. Herpes in the newborn, called neonatal herpes, is extremely rare. Most often, the baby acquires the virus while moving down the birth canal. The newborn is bathed in virus-containing secretions from the mucous membranes of the canal. Herpes enters the newborn's body either through the skin or through the mucous membranes of the mouth, rectum, or genital tract. In rare instances, virus in the mother's blood can cross the placenta, infecting the baby's bloodstream directly. Finally, virus can be picked up during the first month of life when the baby is susceptible to many viruses and bacteria because of an immature immune system. In this case, the baby usually contracts herpes by direct contact with the mother's genital or oral secretions. I have been consulted in instances where a mother with sores on her breast has passed the virus to her infant while breast-feeding. If other household members have an active case of herpes, they can infect the baby by intimate contact.

Q. If I have herpes during pregnancy, can I deliver my baby safely?

A. Yes. But you must advise your doctor of your herpes history so the necessary precautions can be made to ensure a normal delivery. One of my patients, Mrs. Whitmore, neglected to do this. Management of herpes during pregnancy is discussed further in chapter 3.

Q. How do I know if I have genital herpes? If I have it, what should I do?

A. Please read on. Chapter 3 answers those questions.

Genital Herpes:
Saving Your Sanity and Sex Life

Genital herpes has a profound effect on many of its victims until they learn that this disease can be controlled and treated. Discovering how can preserve your sanity and your sex life. Let's meet a married couple and two single adults who confronted the difficulties of diagnosis and the fear of transmitting herpes to a loved one. They satisfactorily resolved—in different ways—their physical and psychological problems.

MELINDA AND JIM: A MARITAL CRISIS

My husband, Jim, and I, both in our mid-twenties, have been happily married for five years. We were college sweethearts, meeting in French class and falling in love—just like a storybook romance. We both graduated with honors, landed good jobs in our respective fields—I'm a teacher, he's an accountant—and married a few months later. I felt blessed that my life seemed so perfect. Until Jim said he might have herpes, and I could be infected, too! The news came at the worst possible time—a few days before our planned second wedding anniversary, to be celebrated as a second honeymoon in the Bahamas.

I had an intuitive feeling that Jim was troubled by something. He began to act very strangely. First he was pensive, then irritable, and finally withdrawn. One night while we were drinking wine by the fire, Jim suddenly started to cry. "Melinda, I think I have VD, and I don't know how I got it. I'm sorry."

I, too, cried. Although I believed Jim, I knew you don't catch venereal disease out of thin air. He wasn't having an affair; I was sure of that because we spent all our free time together. I thought our relationship was even better than when we first married. The source of Jim's VD was a mystery. We decided to consult a doctor together.

We knew our physician quite well. We both had seen him for annual physicals, and he treated me once for strep throat and Jim for an ear infection. We liked him because he was always matter-of-fact and never seemed so busy that he couldn't answer simple questions. But, on this occasion, I sensed he was somewhat uncomfortable because of the nature of the discussion.

Jim's self-diagnosis was correct. He had typical herpes lesions on his penis, enlarged lymph glands, and a slight fever. The doctor also examined me but found no sign of herpes. After our examinations, we sat together in his office. As you can imagine, we both had lots of questions. I felt like crying but somehow kept my composure. I'm sure Jim felt ashamed; he avoided looking me straight in the eyes.

The doctor pulled a medical textbook from his library shelf, appeared to check the index, and opened to the section on viruses. Then he began to read: "Herpes genitalis is an infection commonly marked by recrudescent vesicles."

"Melinda, do you know what that means?" he asked.

"It means the blisters come and go," I replied.

"Exactly, and their reappearance doesn't necessarily follow logic or any set chronological schedule," the doctor said. "And the original infection is not always obvious to the herpes victim."

After the doctor discussed latency with us in more detail, I felt that Jim was, after all, telling me the truth. I knew that he had dated a few women before me—one seriously for quite some time—and that she may have been the source of the virus.

Herpes has not changed our relationship substantially because we've been able to cope with it. Jim's outbreaks are infrequent—maybe once every six months—which I liken to my monthly menstrual periods. I know he's in some discomfort, so I try to be a little more sensitive to his needs. I guess I probably spoil him.

I still think I'm a pretty lucky woman.

JEFF'S STORY: A DIAGNOSTIC DILEMMA

I contracted genital herpes in November 1975—well before the disease reached the front pages of newspapers and patients began streaming into the examining rooms of VD clinics in record numbers. By the time my herpes was correctly diagnosed, I was relieved that it was only herpes and not something more serious, as I had been led to believe.

I was 30 years old, and in very good health—a marathon runner and avid tennis player. I was making plans to relocate from Atlanta to New York City when my problem began. Like most herpes sufferers, I tried to ignore the symptoms at first. I attributed the tightness in my groin to muscle strain from running. When the blisters first appeared on my penis, I became concerned but chose not to seek medical help for several days. "It will pass; no cause for alarm," I said to myself.

The ache worsened. I felt constant discomfort while walking, and I couldn't run. The blisters began to ooze a milky-white pus. The pain intensified. Reluctantly, I decided to see a doctor. Because I didn't have a regular family physician at the time, I contacted an internist I knew casually from my church.

By the time my appointment finally rolled around, the blisters had dried and the scabs were gone. The ache was tolerable. But the doctor could still detect a knot about the size of a pebble in my groin. After the physical, we moved from the examining room to his private office for what he said would be "a little chat." At this point I knew I was in trouble. "Jeff, it's difficult to say what you have, but it's obviously some kind of infection. Your lymph nodes are enlarged, indicating you have a lot of white cells working at something foreign in your system. I can't see any lesions on your penis. You may have had some sort of venereal disease, which as you know can be very contagious. To know for sure and to give you peace of mind, we'll order some tests to see what it is." He outlined the possibilities: syphilis, genital herpes, chancroid, or some strange thing called LGV for lymphogranuloma venereum. He suspected the last.

It would be several days before the results were known. Meantime, the doctor suggested that I notify any women with whom I had recent sexual relations. I shared with him my predicament: I had been involved with two women during the past few months. Each is going to wonder how I got venereal disease since I reasoned that *both* were not carriers of whatever it was I had.

The doctor sympathized with my plight but warned that the potential consequences of some forms of venereal disease are very serious and that even the milder diseases such as herpes could spread easily and contribute to an epidemic. In women, he added, the LGV symptoms are often undetected until the virus has spread to vital parts of the body.

The resulting conversations with my two girl friends were cold and ugly, as you could imagine. One reacted violently—narrowly missing me with a pot as I walked out the door. The other initially refused to see or talk with me until I identified the "other woman." I confessed my infidelity and urged both to contact their gynecologists for treatment.

Lab tests confirmed that I had a high titer (amount) of antibody against herpes simplex and was apparently recuperating from a recent attack of genital herpes. I also had a low titer of antibody against LGV, suggesting an LGV infection in the distant past. Emotionally, I felt fortunate that I had herpes and nothing worse. I was relieved that the mystery was finally solved—even though there were no guarantees for treatment.

The ache in my groin never returned, but I continued to experience blistering every few months for about two years. Each episode seemed to be less painful than the previous bout. I suspect that the stress associated with moving and guilt related to letting two women each believe they were my "one and only" reactivated the latent virus I probably picked up a long time ago.

All in all, herpes was a good learning experience for me. I discovered something about my body and my character. My body has healed, but I will never totally repair the emotional bridges that collapsed with my girl friends. I know now that intimacy means a lot more than sex.

JENNIFER: A VOLUNTARY CELIBATE

I used to like sex a lot. I wasn't a sex fiend or anything like that, but I did enjoy physical relationships with several different men. So when the doctor diagnosed "herpes," I was angry. I blamed myself.

I was 31 years old, with a good job—regional marketing director for a pharmaceutical company—which had a promising future. Most of my knowledge of herpes came from reading advice columns in the newspaper. I never thought it would happen to me.

My herpes was detected during a routine pelvic examination by my gynecologist. When the doctor pointed out tiny blisters in my genital area, I remembered recently having some discomfort during urination.

My work schedule is erratic. As a result, my relationships with men tend to be occasional. I travel a lot on my job and spend the weekends recuperating at home. I do recall feeling quite fatigued about a week after having sexual relations with a new acquaintance. I thought I had caught the flu. When I told my doctor about the new sex partner and the weakness and achiness a week later, she guessed that it was my first attack of genital herpes.

Herpes has had one positive effect on me: it has forced me to reevaluate my sexual behavior. I never associated sex with any kind of commitment. Of course, I didn't go to bed with every man I met. But I believed that single adults, especially those of my age, need to fulfill biological needs, such as sex, just as much as married people.

Because some of my sexual encounters were with casual friends, I have decided to change my life-style. I cannot afford to sleep with a man, give him herpes, and jeopardize his health. I also don't want to get the reputation of being loose with my morality.

I'm not interested in any long-term commitments right now, but that might change if Mr. Wonderful comes along. In the meantime, I've become celibate, at least until doctors find a cure. I know they have a new drug that can treat herpes, but they don't give you any guarantees that the blisters won't return.

I joined a support group for herpes sufferers. I attend infrequently because of my schedule. Sometimes I don't feel that I belong because I think I'm in pretty good control of my life. But I admit that I have occasional feelings of anger, mostly toward myself, because I didn't take better precautions.

THE SEATTLE PROFILE OF GENITAL HERPES

Were Jim, Melinda, Jeff, and Jennifer "typical" herpes victims? To answer this, let's look at a demographic and behavioral study of genital herpes, conducted at the University of Washington Genital Herpes Simplex Virus Clinic in Seattle between 1975 and 1980. More than 600 patients were evaluated in the six-year period. Who fits their patients' profile?

•   The average patient was 27 and had 15.1 years of formal education, which means about three years of college or technical training following high school.

•   Sixty-four percent of the patients were single.

•   In most cases, genital herpes was their first encounter with venereal disease.

•   Sixty-six percent of women and 61 percent of men with first episodes of genital herpes had only one sexual partner during the 30 days before acquisition of the virus, and 39 percent of all patients had a new sexual partner within 30 days of onset.

•   Oral sex was performed within the last two weeks by 48 percent of the patients and 47 percent of the sexual partners.

The Seattle researchers taught us that although some similarities were apparent, their patients were by no means homogeneous. Herpes is a disease primarily, but not exclusively, of young adults. They may, or may not, have many sexual partners. And in most cases, but not every case, herpes was acquired from the most recent sexual partner.

In other words, there is no such a thing as a "classic" case of genital herpes. Genital herpes is not necessarily the mark of sexual promiscuity. You can catch the virus from a single sexual encounter. As herpes spreads throughout the population, the chance of exposure—especially with a new sexual partner—increases. You can become infected if you are married, or if you are single.

DIAGNOSIS CAN BE DIFFICULT

The diagnosis of genital herpes is not always easy, even for an experienced clinician. In many cases the patient has waited until some symptoms have disappeared and sores are healing before seeking medical attention. Other patients are less than candid about their sexual experiences and practices, which handicaps a physician trying to take an accurate medical history. Although genital herpes symptoms are well defined, they can mimic other forms of VD and even nonvenereal skin diseases such as psoriasis. On rare occasions, some of the signs indicate more serious illnesses.

For most victims, genital herpes is their first encounter with venereal disease. As a result, they may ignore the pain until it becomes unbearable. Public health experts agree that many people are not seeking medical attention even with obvious signs of a venereal disease.

For your own well-being and that of others, see a doctor or public health nurse if you notice any of the major signals of herpes. Self-diagnosis by a lay person is unwise and possibly dangerous to one's health. Your doctor has the best chance to make the correct diagnosis when the rash is fresh. If your diagnosis is genital herpes, don't be afraid. Help is available. Ask questions. Knowledge of your disease will give you power over it.

Accurate Diagnosis

In most instances, a physician can make the proper diagnosis based on a medical history, which involves a brief interview to collect details about your physical activities, feelings, and past health, followed by a physical examination. But sometimes the doctor is uncertain. Perhaps your problem is due to trauma or a different kind of venereal disease. Fortunately, doctors have laboratory tools to confirm or deny the presumptive diagnosis. Your doctor may order one or more of the following tests:

• Lesion smear (Tzanck test). A simple scraping of skin or mucosal lesions provides enough cells for a microscopic examination. Following the application of a special stain, the doctor or laboratory technologist is able to look for cells that contain many nuclei: a sign of cell damage resulting from herpes. This test is very similar to a method routinely used for detection of cancer of the female genital tract, called a Pap smear.

- Culture. Many laboratories are equipped to grow the virus from a swab specimen of the patient's sores. In addition to determining whether herpes simplex is present, some labs can distinguish between type 1 and type 2. Knowing the virus type is helpful in predicting frequency of recurrences. Culture tests can also diagnose other diseases such as chancroid that may be responsible for venereal sores.

- Blood sample. Presence of specific antibodies, protein molecules made by certain white blood cells, indicates whether you have experienced a herpes attack at any time in the past. Some laboratories can tell if you have antibody against herpes simplex type 1 or type 2.

- One-day herpes test. Kits employing any of the above methods are being marketed as rapid tests.

PRIMARY (FIRST) INFECTIONS

The incubation period for primary genital herpes averages six days but has been reported to be as short as one day and as long as a month and a half. In 30 percent of all cases, patients do not recognize their primary herpes attack because the symptoms are so mild. But the majority report that their first outbreak is the most painful, the most severe, and lasts the longest, an average of 14 to 17 days.

Symptoms

- Malaise. A feeling of general discomfort or uneasiness is often the first sign of the infection. Malaise is especially noticeable if you are in general good health, fit, and rarely feel "under the weather."

- Muscle aches. You may experience generalized achiness, particularly of large muscles, reminiscent of the flu.

- Fever. About one-third of victims report fever that may be accompanied by shaking chills or night sweats. Fever sometimes precedes the rash.

- Rash. Doctors refer to all forms of herpes rash as "lesions." In men, lesions most often occur on the head or shaft of the penis. In women, lesions generally surface on the external parts of the genitals: the vulva or clitoris. Lesions are commonly found on the cervix, but detection requires a pelvic examination by the physician. Herpes lesions may also appear near the genitals on the buttocks, thighs, and in the rectal area (especially in those performing oral-rectal or genital-rectal sex).

The rash of herpes evolves as follows: papules (small lumps) and

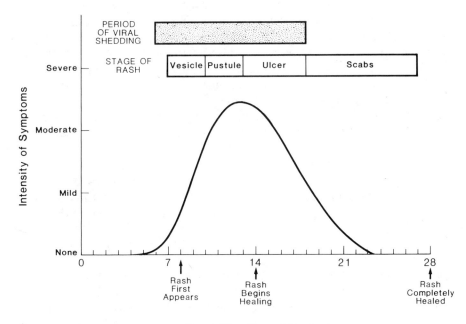

The typical course of primary genital herpes.

vesicles (blisters) surrounded by reddened, swollen tissue develop on the skin or mucous membranes of the genitals. Papules quickly turn into vesicles or disappear. Vesicles tend to be large and numerous in first episodes of genital herpes but may be as small as a pencil point in mild cases. New lesions may continue to form for as long as a week. New vesicles contain clear fluid that becomes cloudy as white cells enter to form pus. The lesions are now termed, appropriately, pustules. Pustules pop within a week, leaving shallow raw areas of skin or mucous membranes called ulcers. Skin ulcers crust, and the crusts or scabs fall off when healing is complete. Ulcers on mucous membranes heal from the outside in, usually without scabbing.

• Pain. When skin or mucous membranes in your genital area are damaged by herpes simplex, tiny nerve endings are stimulated and you feel pain. Pain associated with genital herpes can be intense. Pain may be due to virions irritating the nerves as they migrate along nerve fibers from your genitals toward the nerve cell bodies located near the spine. Any place the rash is present may be painful, especially the rectum.

• Itching. Think of pain as a continuum. Itchiness is the mildest sort of pain. As herpes simplex destroys healthy cells, damaged fragments of the cells are released, which results in inflammation of surrounding tissues. The itchy feeling indicates mild damage to the skin or mucous membranes. Itching is common when lesions start and also when lesions heal. Some patients experience tingling or an itchy sensation in their genital area after the rash heals. This may result from virions migrating from the genitals along nerve pathways and stimulating the nerves to tingle in the process.

• Painful urination. The urethra is a mucous membrane tube through which urine flows from the bladder. Herpes simplex damages the cells of the urethra, forming tiny blisters that break open, leaving the canal sensitive. A few victims have such pain they are unable to urinate and require catheterization in order to void.

• Painful intercourse. The blisters are sensitive to any kind of touch, especially intercourse. This may be the first indication of herpes, particularly for women whose blisters are deep in the vaginal canal and unseen during self-examination.

• Swollen and tender inguinal (groin) lymph glands. Glands are usually sensitive and sometimes painful. You may feel a dull ache, pressure, or throbbing. Don't be alarmed if you feel a pebble or a knot! This almost never means a cancerous tumor. The lymph glands enlarge because they are packed with white blood cells trying to fight off the virus. Another term for lymph gland is lymph node—node literally means a knot.

• Headache and stiff neck. About one-fourth of herpes patients report such symptoms during first attacks. These are more common in women. They may be signs that the virus has invaded the body's central nervous system to produce inflammation of the coverings of the brain and spinal cord called meninges.

The severity of all these symptoms varies greatly. In general, women are sicker than men. Some victims are hardly aware of their infection, whereas others are sick enough to be bedridden or hospitalized for a week or more.

RECURRENCES

During our primary herpes attack, viral particles wend their way from the genital area along nerve pathways to ganglia (collections of nerve cell bodies) near the base or sacral area of our spine. The virions become dormant inside neurons (nerve cells). Herpes never surfaces again in some patients, but the majority suffer recurrences when the virions periodically awaken and travel back down nerve pathways to the genitals.

Many patients suffering recurrent episodes say they actually feel an attack is coming on because of a peculiar sensation near the site of original infection. The feeling has been described as tingling, itching, burning, numbness, or pain. Some patients also have headaches. These symptoms are referred to as the prodrome, a medical term for a group of symptoms indicating the onset of disease. The prodrome precedes the actual outbreak of blisters by at least several hours, and possibly as long as two days according to some patients. Think of the prodrome as a warning signal that distress is near. In a way, your body is sending an SOS.

Most patients report fewer blisters during recurrent attacks. In men and women the recurrent blisters tend to appear at the original site of infection. Glandular swelling is less pronounced. Fever and headaches may accompany each recurrence.

HELP, a national organization of herpes victims based in California, surveyed 7500 members in October 1979 to collect information on herpes diagnosis, frequency of recurrence, and characteristics of the members. Approximately half of the men and women polled returned the questionnaire. Although this method of gathering scientific data involved the inherent problem of self-selectivity and therefore skewed

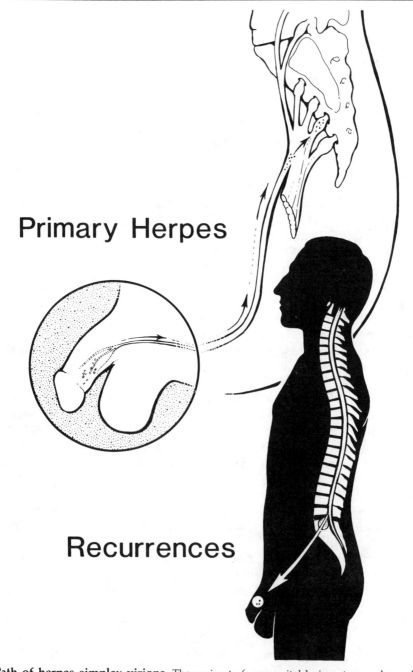

Primary Herpes

Recurrences

Path of herpes simplex virions. They migrate from genital lesions to sacral ganglia during primary herpes and from the ganglia back to the skin during recurrences.

the results, the survey offers insight into the severity and frequency of recurrences.

HELP reported that 8.8 percent of the patients had no recurrences or only one. Approximately one-fourth of the respondents said they experienced two to four attacks a year. Two-thirds had five or more episodes a year. A small group of about 5 percent reported chronic herpes, meaning their genital herpes infections were almost always present.

On first glance, the HELP survey would seem alarming to new sufferers of the disease because of the preponderance of chronic and persistent cases. But we must remember that highly motivated individuals with difficult herpes are likely to join HELP and respond to the questionnaires. As indicated earlier, most clinicians and patients report that recurrences become less frequent and less intense as time passes.

What Triggers a Recurrence?

Medical science still lacks a definitive answer to the most puzzling question about genital herpes. The unpredictability of recurrence aggravates the anxiety felt by some patients. Health professionals and patients have identified several "triggers" that seem to awaken the hibernating virus and spur it into new activity. The most common triggers are emotional stress, lack of sleep, fever, sexual intercourse, masturbation, friction from tight-fitting clothes, and extended exposure to the sun and wind.

But many patients say they are certain that their herpes reactivates for no apparent reason. They don't feel stressed. They abstain from sexual intercourse. They appear healthy, both mentally and physically. How do we explain recurrences in these individuals?

Studies at the University of Minnesota Chronobiology Laboratory were among the first to show that biological rhythms can influence susceptibility to disease, response to therapy, and performance in both mental and physical testing. Each of us has a timing device within our bodies called the biologic clock. This clock regulates the ebb and flow of our daily lives. Although we are not conscious that the clock is ticking, it governs our habit patterns—some of us are morning people, some night owls; some productive on Mondays, some gloomy on Fridays.

The chronobiology of herpes recurrence is theoretical. To my knowledge, no scientist has specifically studied herpes recurrence from the chronobiologic viewpoint. But I speculate the biological cycle runs like this:

Hormones are powerful substances that affect every organ and system in the body. Their activity is regulated by the biologic clock. One group of hormones, called steroids, are immunosuppressive. They exert many effects on our immune system, including a decrease in the number of lymphocytes circulating in our bloodstream. In the proper context, the biologic clock could signal an outbreak of genital herpes by making steroid activity high, resulting in lowered immunity. The cell climate would be just right for herpes simplex to wake up and proceed down the nerve pathways to cause another outbreak.

Why do recurrent episodes diminish over time? We don't know for sure. One possible explanation can be given by using the analogy of garden seeds. If you buy fresh seeds and plant them in your garden right away, almost all will sprout. But if you leave the seeds in their packet for two years before planting, perhaps only half of them will grow. The longer the seeds remain in their packet, the less able they are to germinate. Herpes virions in the nerve ganglia may be like seeds in their packet. If the virions aren't "triggered" to erupt in the first season, they are less likely to sprout in the following seasons.

Confirming this theory would require a long-term study of untreated patients. Because of new and effective antiviral therapies, it's doubtful that such a study will ever be undertaken.

MANAGING YOUR DISEASE

"Herpes is forever" suggests a lifelong illness—an existence of celibacy, a psyche scarred by disease. "Forever" also conveys the impression that nothing can be done to manage the disease or cope with physical and emotional consequences. But genital herpes is not forever, even if the virus remains in your system. You *can* manage herpes. I suggest the following program.

Learn about the Disease

Obtain accurate medical information about herpes. In the process, you will learn a lot about the human body and its vast resources of resistance. The disease is much less intimidating when you learn the facts. Knowledge also provides a sense of control. If you know how to recognize symptoms of recurrence, you may be able to rearrange your routine to accommodate the disease without letting it interfere with your normal life-style.

Take Care of Yourself

Proper nutrition, exercise, relaxation, and sleep all result in a state of general well-being. There is no scientific evidence that proves a certain diet will keep you herpes-free. However, good nutrition and physical exercise do contribute to a healthy body and a positive sense about yourself. There are no guarantees that you will avoid recurrences, but you will certainly reap other benefits.

Because you may have recurrences despite taking care of yourself, select a personal physician who sees you regularly. You will be more comfortable discussing personal matters with someone you trust. Your doctor will appreciate more readily your physical changes because he or she has seen and recorded all previous findings.

Although stress reduction hasn't been proven to reduce the number of recurrences, herpes sufferers have told me that an important factor triggering recurrences is stress. We live in a stressful world— pressure to get "A's," to earn more money, to be the "first." Being good to yourself is an effective way to reduce stress. Dr. Wayne Dyer, author of many common sense self-help books, puts it best in *Your Erroneous Zones*:

> *You may have a social disease, one that will not go away with a simple injection. You are quite possibly infected with the sepsis of low-esteem, and the only known cure is a massive dose of self-love. But perhaps, like many in our society, you've grown up with the idea that loving yourself is wrong. Think of others, society tells us. Love thy neighbor, the church admonishes. What nobody seems to remember is love thyself, and yet that is precisely what you're going to have to learn to do if you are to achieve present-moment happiness.*

My advice is to pamper yourself. Why not take a few hours off one afternoon to watch a movie you've been dying to see? Or visit a museum. Do whatever you find enjoyable. Some firms permit the use of wildcard vacation days to allow employees to recharge their batteries. If wildcard days are available, take them. Physicist Albert Einstein was sometimes seen ambling down Nassau Street in Princeton, New Jersey, licking a doubledip ice cream cone! Einstein knew how to escape his "think tank" and indulge himself without being self-conscious.

Express Your Feelings

We all have emotions that if held within ourselves too long can cause physical harm. The key is to let them out: cry, beat a pillow, paint, talk to a friend, join a support group. If you are deeply troubled, obtain professional counseling. Remember, the anguish eventually will pass. Better days are ahead. You will recover. Look for the gift in the crisis. You can learn about intimacy, sex, illness, your body.

Follow These Tips

• See a doctor. Physicians now have specific therapy called acyclovir (brand name Zovirax) that will help you. The ointment form of the drug is applied three to five times a day, using a glove or finger cot. Acyclovir pills, when available, will be useful if your sores are internal. Intravenous acyclovir is also available and works if your problem is severe enough to require hospitalization. For more information on acyclovir, see chapter 9.

• Practice good hygiene. Keep herpes lesions clean by washing with warm, soapy water, then rinsing. Dry carefully and thoroughly by patting involved areas, or use a hair dryer at a low setting. Rough rubbing may burst the sores and cause virus to spread, producing inflammation and more discomfort.

• Don't touch, pick, or puncture blisters. The fluid contains millions of tiny infectious virions. Their release will spread infection and delay healing.

• Wash your hands more frequently than usual. Don't touch your eyes if virus is active because herpes can infect them.

• Keep lesions dry by applying drying agents like talcum powder, corn starch, or a similar substance recommended by your physician.

• Sleep in the nude, allowing air naturally to dry the vesicles.

• Wear loose-fitting, 100 percent cotton undergarments. Avoid acrylics and tight-fitting pants.

• If urination is painful, relieve yourself in a tub full of warm water.

• Apply ice or an icepack for severe pain. Cold compresses do *not* kill virus, as some books have suggested, but your discomfort may be minimized.

• Try a sitz bath. Add one tablespoon of salt per quart of warm water to a basin, and soak your genitals for five to ten minutes. This may be repeated two to three times daily.

• Avoid prolonged or frequent bathing and keep the water tepid. Hot water may aggravate your genital sores.
• Try a numbing anesthetic ointment.
• Aspirin may relieve pain and headache.
• Minimize stress. Try relaxation exercises.
• Women beginning at age 18 should have regular Pap smears at least once a year. A Pap smear can diagnose recurrent herpes as well as signal the advent of genital tract cancer. Later in this chapter, I'll discuss the tenuous relationship between herpes and genital cancer.

Where to Go for Additional Help

1. Write to HELP (which stands for Herpetics Engaged in Living Productively), sponsored by the American Social Health Organization, P.O. Box 100, Palo Alto, California 94302. HELP publishes a quarterly newsletter, "The Helper," filled with the latest results of proven treatments and advice on coping. The national headquarters can provide information about local chapters that offer educational and counseling services.

2. Call the National VD Hotline for answers to your questions (1–800–227–8922).

3. Your city or state public health department may sponsor a special infectious disease clinic. Call and find out what's available.

4. Inquire about support groups that may have been organized through your church, synagogue, or school.

5. Some patients have benefited most from private consultation with a clinical psychologist.

THE PSYCHOLOGICAL DIMENSION OF HERPES

In *The Scarlet Letter*, an American classic, author Nathaniel Hawthorne writes an intense, tragic story of the psychological effects of adultery on four people, including Hester Prynne, who was forced to wear a scarlet "A" over her heart. Although ostracized and persecuted in her New England village, Hester feels no shame for her act and refuses to wear her "A" in disgrace. Instead, she decorates the letter with gold thread.

The social stigma of genital herpes has been likened to the modern day scarlet letter. The lesson that Hawthorne told in 1850 may also apply today. Hester Prynne survived ridicule, maintained her self-respect, and became a stronger person in the end.

Brad's Story

I've had herpes for about seven years now. Until the attacks stopped a year ago, I suffered recurrences every three months. Perhaps the virus has gone into remission. My wife, Laurie, has an outbreak once every six months. Although we took the suggested precautions—no sex when sores were evident, and I wore a condom for a week after the sores were completely healed—she caught the virus about six months after we were married.

We've both adjusted pretty well to the problem. Part of that, I'm sure, is due to the strength of our marriage. But we both agree that this emotion-suicide-guilt complex issue is way out of proportion to the reality of the problem.

I know a lot has been written about the emotional crisis some people face, but I just don't believe that many people suffer emotional breakdowns because of it. Sure, herpes is annoying and sometimes painful. But so is the flu. I used to think of herpes as having an attack of the flu three or four times a year. You accept it, work through it, and get better. You know you're going to be well again.

Jill's Story

When I caught herpes, I thought I was the unluckiest person in the world. It was my first sexual encounter and the relationship fell apart soon afterward. When I became ill, I was alone, away from home at college, with no close friends. I finally confided in my roommate, who commented, "Don't be so upset. There are worse things that could happen to you. Just think about all the people with cancer or heart disease."

I went home for a holiday and, by coincidence, the dinner conversation focused on herpes. My parents had seen some television special about herpes and said they were disgusted to hear that so many unmarried people were having sex. Mom said, "Those girls are just sluts." I was almost ready to ask my parents for some support and she goes and says that. I quietly slipped off to my room and cried.

After returning to school, I talked with a counselor who was most supportive. She put it all in perspective. I doubt that I will ever tell my parents, but that doesn't seem important any longer. I know the herpes will probably go away. I plan to begin my sex life anew. But the next time, I'm going to ask my lover a few questions.

Coping with Your Disease

While most men and women may cope with herpes as Brad and his wife did simply by learning its cause and physical progression, others such as Jill may need counseling—from either a friend or a professional—to work through feelings of anger, blame, shame, and guilt.

Counselors emphasize that emotions are a normal and potentially positive psychological reaction to a health crisis. Although not everyone responds in the same way, many people go through five identifiable stages, suggests Irene Bugge, PhD, a clinical psychologist at the University of Minnesota student health service who has worked with young adults both individually and in group settings. She offers the following model to help explain emotional response to the disease:

Denial. After the doctor confirms the herpes diagnosis, you may react with disbelief: "I can't have herpes," you say. "There must be some mistake." When the doctor advises a course of treatment, you become numb. "This must be happening to someone else." Denial is a common human response to the onset of the disease. We simply refuse to accept that our health has been impaired and that our normal life-style must change. If you get stuck at the denial stage, you may fail to obtain the necessary medical attention that you need or refuse to comply with the right treatment plan. You may infect others because of your unwillingness to believe that you have herpes.

Depression. As the reality of the diagnosis sinks in, depression, self-pity, and despair may envelop you. You are likely to ask, "Why me? Why did I get herpes?" You may wonder if you will ever have a normal sex life. You may feel like a leper. You may ask yourself if there is any reason to go on living. Becoming entrenched in the depression stage may mean that you spend a significant portion of your time alone and engaged in self-pity. A few do something extreme and give up, drop out, even consider suicide.

Shame/Guilt. You may intensify your feelings of depression by concluding that you deserved to get herpes, that herpes is the price you must pay for "free love." Accepting the social stigma attached to herpes, you decide not to tell anyone. "I can't tell my parents. What will my friends think of me if I tell them?" You may feel very alone—shamefully alone with this disease. If you can't overcome your feelings of shame and guilt, you may brand yourself an outcast and not reach out to draw support from others.

Anger. The self-blaming may be followed by feelings of anger and resentment directed toward others. You feel animosity toward the medical profession for not having a cure. You become angry at the person who gave you herpes, and if you hold onto that feeling you may waste your time plotting revenge. Dr. Bugge says: "There is considerable energy in anger, and this feeling can serve as a catalyst to head in a different direction. You may become committed to not spreading the disease to others. Or you may invest some of your energy to help others with this disease. For example, you might offer to talk with others newly diagnosed with herpes, or assist in creation of a support group."

Acceptance. Beyond the shock and denial, the depression and self-blame, beyond the anger, you are likely to come to accept the fact that you have genital herpes. You are now ready to ask yourself, "Will I let this disease dominate my life? Of course not." Psychologists suggest that once you have accepted your herpes, there's a way to grow and mature from the experience. Ask yourself, "Have I grown in some ways, learned some things about myself, sex, intimacy, from this experience? Can these events enhance my life? Can I share them with others?"

These stages are not linear. Patients do not automatically progress from the first through fifth stages, finally resolving their troubles after reaching "acceptance." Most likely, you will circle back through all these feelings at different times. For example, after you've had herpes for a while, you will meet someone special, someone with whom you would really like to develop a close and intimate relationship. You know you must talk with this person about herpes. You'll probably matriculate through the entire spectrum of emotions before you talk with him or her.

Recognize that each and every one of these feelings is natural and legitimate. However, if you become stuck for a prolonged period at any one of the first four stages, your enjoyment of life may be compromised. You could even hurt others.

TELLING A LOVED ONE ABOUT HERPES

There are countless successful approaches to telling a friend that you have genital herpes. Of course, you don't have to say anything at all about herpes unless you are contemplating a sexual relationship. But I advise you to tell before rather than after the fact.

What patients fear most is being rejected after revealing their diagnosis. If the information about genital herpes is relayed thoughtfully, calmly, and honestly, I believe most potential sex partners will react with sensitivity to your condition. Familiarize yourself with the medical facts so that you can answer questions accurately. I suggest that your approach be positive: herpes is preventable, manageable, and treatable. Remember, an attack of genital herpes doesn't mean that you have been sexually promiscuous. Thousands have acquired the disease from one encounter. Even monogamous couples have suffered genital herpes many years after a faithful marriage because of the unpredictability and frequency of recurrences.

An important reason to talk openly about genital herpes is the possibility of two serious complications—one that can affect your sex partner directly and the other that can strike his or her offspring. Your partner could contract chronic herpes—herpes that never goes away completely. I estimate this risk to be one in a thousand, but even that slight probability can be reduced further by early treatment. The more serious complication is neonatal herpes.

HERPES IN THE NEWBORN

Neonatal herpes is a rare complication of genital herpes. Babies tend to be sicker if their mothers suffer primary rather than recurrent herpes during pregnancy. Here are two examples illustrating possible consequences of a disease that strikes approximately one in 7,500 infants.

Brenda's Story

Christine Sorenson attended prenatal classes at the county hospital. She showed no visible symptoms of genital herpes during her regular physical examinations. After 37 weeks of pregnancy she went into premature labor and delivered a tiny girl weighing five pounds. The infant, who was named Brenda, appeared normal in the delivery room, but when she was transferred to the nursery a pediatric resident observed rapid breathing and red spots on her back. She was therefore moved to the neonatal intensive care unit. A chest X ray revealed pneumonia, and the doctor prescribed antibiotics.

Within a few hours the red spots became enlarged and filled with fluid. They were scraped for microscopic examination and culture. Because giant cells typical of herpes were not seen under the microscope, the viral diagnosis remained in doubt. During the next two days the baby's pneumonia worsened, her liver enlarged, and she had the first of many seizures. Then, the director of the Virology Lab at the Health Department called to report that the culture was growing herpes simplex. The diagnosis was no longer in doubt—Brenda had neonatal herpes. She was started on a drug called cytarabine that offered some promise of being effective against herpes. The baby slowly improved over the next several weeks, but it was clear to the neonatologists that she had sustained serious brain damage. The seizures continued, her general muscle strength was poor, and her suck remained weak.

The mother, Christine, was emotionally traumatized by her baby's illness. She was only 18, single, and without a permanent job. The father, who had been involved in several sexual affairs during the pregnancy, abandoned her near the time of delivery. Because of her financial and marital status, Christine tentatively had decided to give the baby up for adoption—until she grasped the severity of her baby's illness. As Brenda's condition deteriorated, the mother's guilt became obvious as she spent more and more time in the nursery. Christine's mood changes were dramatic, ranging from numbness one day to hysteria the next. A hospital social worker and a psychologist intervened to help Christine accept the fact that her baby would require continuous care by medical professionals.

When she was three months old the baby's condition stabilized and she was transferred to a permanent home for brain-damaged children. Brenda, born in 1970, is severely retarded and remains institutionalized to this day. The young mother required several years of counseling before she was finally able to cope with her guilt.

Mary's Cesarean Section

Mary, age 20, has recurrent genital herpes. When she became pregnant for the first time, she told her doctor about her herpes history immediately. Recognizing the potential risk of neonatal herpes, Mary's obstetrician examined her frequently and took genital tract cultures weekly during her last trimester. At 38 weeks of pregnancy, one of Mary's vaginal specimens contained herpes, although she had no genital sores at the time. A week later Mary felt a sudden intense urgency to void. Rushing to the bathroom, she discharged a large amount of straw-colored fluid. Alarmed, she called her doctor's office for advice.

"Mary, your membranes have ruptured," the nurse told her. "Are you having regular contractions?

"No."

"Well, in any case, you had better come to the hospital. I'll notify the doctor on call."

Mary was admitted and two hours later taken to the operating room where baby Aaron was born by cesarean section. Aaron weighed seven pounds five ounces. He breast fed well, did beautifully in the newborn nursery, and went home when his mother was discharged from the hospital eight days later. When I last saw Aaron he was a normal six-month-old boy. Mary told me that he has never had any sign of herpes.

Comment: If a woman has genital herpes sores or evidence by laboratory tests that herpes is active in the last few weeks of pregnancy, most doctors will perform an elective cesarean section before active labor begins. The cesarean section prevents the baby from coming in contact with herpes during passage through the vagina. If the baby is delivered through an infected birth canal, the risk of neonatal herpes is estimated to be 2 percent. In patients with active herpes whose membranes rupture spontaneously, an emergency cesarean section usually is performed within four hours, before the virus has had a chance to ascend directly into the uterus to infect the infant. A cesarean section is unnecessary if genital herpes is inactive as determined by a physician at the time the membranes rupture.

Neonatal Herpes in Perspective

These two stories about the rare disease neonatal herpes contain several common elements. Both mothers fit the profile of women whose babies develop neonatal herpes. They were young, apparently healthy, had no symptoms of herpes during their pregnancies, and were having their first babies. Then why were the outcomes so drastically different?

Brenda was born in 1970 before many doctors appreciated the urgency of early diagnosis. She was premature, and such infants have more trouble coping with herpes than full-term babies. Finally, the experimental drug she received was later shown to be ineffective against newborn herpes infections.

In contrast, Aaron was born in 1983, a time of heightened awareness of the consequences of neonatal herpes. A doctor quickly made the diagnosis of active herpes in Aaron's mother and delivered him by cesarean section. Either the cesarean section protected Aaron from becoming infected, or his immune system destroyed the virus before it could spread. Full-term, normal-sized infants like Aaron and Jonathan (whose story was detailed in chapter 2) seem more resistant to herpes, probably because their immune systems are more fully developed than those of prematurely born infants like Brenda.

Surprisingly, some babies survived neonatal herpes before the advent of effective antiherpes therapy and grew to live very normal lives. I have cared for two such children. Medical science cannot explain exactly why virus devastates one baby while sparing another. The immune system, so important in our defense against herpesviruses, can handle the virus in some babies without the aid of antiviral drugs.

What can be done to minimize the chances of a disaster such as Brenda's?

• Tell your doctor, just as Mary did, if you or your partner have a history of genital herpes. Your doctor will examine you and may take swab specimens from your genital tract during your last month of pregnancy to look for herpes.

• If you have genital sores or if the specimens show that herpes is present at or near the time of delivery, special precautions will be taken. First, your baby probably will be delivered by cesarean section. Second, some form of isolation will be used for you and your baby because there is a slight chance that other babies might catch the virus. Once your baby leaves the hospital, special isolation precautions are not necessary. Newborns with herpes are a risk only to other newborns.

• Abstain from kissing and sexual intercourse near the time of delivery if you or your partner have oral or genital lesions. If you are not willing to abstain from sex, the male should wear a condom. Neonates have contracted serious herpes infections from their mother's sexual partner very near the time of delivery.

• Your baby should not be fondled or kissed by anyone with oral herpes until the herpetic rash has completely healed. This is especially important when infants are less than a month old. After that time the risk of neonatal herpes is essentially gone.

• You may breast-feed your baby if you have oral or genital herpes provided you wear a fresh gown and mask. You should not breast feed, however, if you have herpes lesions on your breasts.

HERPES AND GENITAL CANCER

Part of the herpes hysteria comes from fear of cancer. Beginning in 1968, a series of studies headed by scientists from Atlanta and Houston indicated that women with cervical cancer had a higher prevalence of herpes antibody and higher titers of antibody than did noncancerous women. These studies often have been cited as evidence for a herpes-cancer link. But the investigations were incomplete, lacking uniformity in selection of subjects and appropriate controls. A direct cause-effect relationship between herpes and cancer was not proved. In fact, many of the women with cancer had no sign of herpes. Because of inconclusive data, scientists have hemmed and hawed for years about the role of herpes in cancer. Thanks to recent research reports, we can now say with certainty that **herpes simplex by itself does not cause genital cancer.**

Dr. Harald zur Hausen of the University of Freiburg, a leading West German authority on this subject, commented at the International Symposium on Medical Virology in Anaheim, California, on October 20, 1983, that carefully planned studies are not substantiating a direct link between herpes and cancer of the cervix.

Yet a relationship between sexual activity and genital cancer has been appreciated for more than a century. In 1842, a landmark article was published in an Italian medical journal by Dr. Rigoni-Stern. Analyzing the vital statistics of Verona, Italy, between 1760 and 1839, he observed that cancers of the uterus (likely most were cancer of the cervix) were rare among unmarried women and cloistered nuns compared with married women and widows. Rigoni-Stern postulated that cervical cancers were somehow linked to sexual activity. Epidemiologic studies in the United States performed nearly 125 years later have supported his incisive observation. Women with cervical cancer tend to be younger at first intercourse and have more sex partners than matched controls without cervical cancer.

Why would the duration of sexual activity and the multiplicity of partners play a role in cervical cancer? Abundant circumstantial evidence suggests that many cancers result from long-term irritation of our tissues. Supporting data include prevalence of skin cancer in persons with excessive sun exposure, and lung cancers in coal miners and smokers who repeatedly inhale foreign substances. The incubation period for most cancers is very long, as reflected by the higher risk of cancer in the elderly.

With these facts in mind, it's easy to understand the association of intercourse and cervical cancer. Secretions induced by sexual activity may produce tissue inflammation because they contain foreign cells and infectious organisms. Having many sexual partners means greater exposure to more and more irritants, of which herpes simplex is only one.

The cancerous potential of these inflammatory agents is additive. This explains why some studies have linked the age at first intercourse with genital cancer. The earlier the exposure to genital irritants, the longer the period of irritation during one's lifetime. Eventually, the threshhold for cancerous growth is reached.

In summary, I believe that genital cancer, including cancer of the cervix and vulva in women and penile cancer in men, is related to multiple irritants that result from sexual promiscuity. Frequent sex with one partner is not a problem. The association between herpes and genital cancer most likely stems from the positive correlation between herpes and having many sex partners. In the Seattle Profile of Genital Herpes, the average number of sexual partners before acquisition of genital herpes was 8.8 for women and 32.8 for men.

QUESTIONS FROM GENITAL HERPES SUFFERERS

Q. Who gets genital herpes?

A. The majority of herpes victims attending VD clinics are young, sexually active, single, and well educated. Of course, others may catch the virus. But epidemiologic studies so far have found genital herpes to be most prevalent in this group.

Q. I have blisters on my genitals. Do I have herpes?

A. Although herpes commonly causes genital blisters, other diseases can do this as well. You should see a medical doctor or a public health nurse at a clinic to confirm or refute your suspicions of genital herpes.

Q. How can I protect my partner?

A. Genital herpes is transmitted through person-to-person contact, most frequently during sexual intercourse. Abstaining from sexual contact when sores are active is the most important thing you can do to prevent spread. This includes kissing if you have active oral lesions. Because both men and women can have herpes simplex in their genital area or mouth without showing visible signs, it is absolutely impossible to totally protect a sexual partner from contracting the disease. Therefore, a frank discussion is a must in any long-term relationship where one partner has the virus. A condom offers some protection, but the shield is not 100 percent effective.

Q. Why does herpes recur?

A. All human herpesviruses are able to enter the cells of our body and persist there in a latent or sleeping state. Genital herpes is no exception. It recurs because the sleeping virus is awakened by some stimulus and migrates down nerve pathways to the genitals.

Q. How can I reduce my chances of recurrence?

A. Patients have told me over and over again that the single most important way to limit recurrences is to minimize stress. Stress reduction can be achieved by engaging in a hobby, exercising, or seeking emotional support from friends or special counseling groups. Divert attention from herpes to something else. Take care of your body, and it will be good to you. Sleep, exercise, proper diet. They all matter.

Q. Will genital herpes lead to cancer?

A. The bulk of scientific evidence indicates that herpes simplex by itself does not cause cancer. Herpes is probably one of many irritants contributing to genital cancer in men and women. All women 18 years of age and older—whether they have herpes or not—should have Pap smears at least yearly to diagnose genital tract cancer, which can be eradicated if detected early. Men or women with genital sores that do not heal should be checked by their doctor.

Q. Will herpes jeopardize my newborn baby?

A. Women with genital herpes can have perfectly normal, healthy, happy babies. You must tell your doctor if you or your partner ever had genital herpes so that your pregnancy can be managed appropriately. Both obstetricians and pediatricians are alert to proper care of this rare but potentially serious complication.

Q. Where can I go for emotional support?

A. A national organization called HELP has branches throughout the country which offer group discussion. The address of their headquarters is given earlier in the chapter. Of course, you may consider individual or group counseling. Services may be available through your college, community clinic, hospital, or a physician referral.

Q. Can herpes be treated?

A. Yes. We now have specific therapies to kill the virus. I also have suggested tips that the patient can use to control recurrent episodes and minimize the pain and emotional trauma. These are discussed earlier in this chapter.

Q. Can herpes be cured?

A. We're tired of hearing the trite phrase "herpes is forever," implying endless infection and suffering. Now we know it isn't true. Many patients experience fewer recurrences over time. Furthermore, a herpes cure already may have been found for some patients with genital herpes. See the story in chapter 9.

Herpes without Sex:
From Cold Sores to Encephalitis

The most common herpes infections are acquired without engaging in sex. We usually catch cold sores during childhood through daily contact with other children. Cold sores are the typical manifestation of herpes simplex virus type 1, which also causes infections of the eyes, fingers, and brain. But the herpes simplex story is not simple. Herpes simplex type 2 can cause cold sores too, and about 15 percent of genital herpes is due to type 1. Both types threaten patients with weakened immunity, just when they seem to be winning their battle against transplant rejection or cancer.

COLD SORES

Because cold sores are hard to hide and the blisters tend to recur, they're the most common form of herpes that we see today. Here are four brief stories from people who suffer from cold sores, also known as oral herpes or herpes labialis.

Larry: I've lived with cold sores since I was about six. I come from a very expressive family with lots of hugging and kissing. I probably caught them from Mom; she still continues to have lots of problems. My sisters caught them too, but I'm the only one with outbreaks every month or so. My cold sores are quite painful and annoying, lasting about 10 days. I know exactly when they're going to happen. The lip tingles, then burns, then the blister pops. It's most likely to occur after I've been in the sun, but I get them in cold weather too.

Joyce: I know exactly when my blister problem began—in Ft. Lauderdale, 1977—and the culprit was my ex-boyfriend. I knew he had cold sores, but, what can I say, I got lost in a moment of passion and kissed him. What a mistake! I had terrible problems while living down there, but now that I'm in Chicago I have outbreaks only a few times a year. I get them in the summer while sailing and in the winter while skiing.

I recall one strange occurrence after I was up all night going through an emotional fit.

Doug: As a landscape architect, I spend a lot of time outdoors during all sorts of weather, surveying property and directing construction crews. If it wasn't for my Chap Stick, I'm certain I would suffer frequent outbreaks since I often feel a strange sensation, kind of like itching, on the lip. I keep my lips covered, even when I don't expect a problem, just for safety. The few times that I failed to use lip ice I ended up with blisters. I'm 29 now. I can't remember when I had my first attack, but it was years ago, probably as a teenager. I was always self-conscious about the blisters. I was even afraid to ask girls for dates because my sores were so unsightly. I'm still embarrassed by my outbreaks.

Susan: I have recurrences only when I come down with a fever—unless I'm pregnant, when I get an attack every month. The doctor says the emotional stress and bodily changes during pregnancy cause the blisters. I've had three children, and it happened every time.

Larry, Joyce, Doug, and Susan all suffer from recurrent herpes lesions of the mouth and lips, a condition that plagues approximately 30 million Americans. If you are lucky enough to be free of cold sores, or fever blisters, you probably harbor the virus within your body anyway—most of us do.

Lesions of the lips and perioral area (around the mouth) look and feel like more of a threat to one's health than they actually are. The sores erupt between 12 and 36 hours after exposure to an environmental, physical, or emotional stimulus. Before blistering, there is a tingling, burning, or itchy feeling of the lips or mouth. The blisters may turn into shallow ulcers but rarely scar. Lesions improve within a few days, but the period of contagiousness extends until the lesions are completely healed, typically a week or slightly longer.

If you look at a developing cold sore under the microscope, you see that the virus-infected skin cells enlarge. Next, the cells behave like social creatures: their outer membranes touch and fuse, something normal cells never do. Once cells fuse, viruses can hop from cell to cell without exposure to their adversaries, the white cells and antibodies of our immune defense. All this cellular socializing results in the formation of a giant cell—many skin cells unite, losing their individual integrity altogether.

How Oral Herpes Is Defined

Doctors often refer to herpes of the lips and mouth as "oral herpes," to distinguish this entity from genital herpes or herpes in the eye. In medical parlance, herpes limited to the lips is called herpes labialis, whereas herpes of the mouth and gums is herpes gingivostomatitis. Recurrent oral herpes is much more common on the lips than inside the mouth, whereas the opposite is true for primary oral herpes.

How Oral Herpes Spreads

Oral herpes infections, like genital herpes, can be spread only by close person-to-person contact. Toddlers are especially prone to catching the virus because they are frequently kissed by parents, siblings, and playmates. The most common period of our lives for catching infections of all sorts is between six months and four years of age.

We all love to cuddle small children. Few parents would ever think of asking someone if they have a history of cold sores before allowing them to kiss a child. But, as mentioned in chapter 3, there's a particular risk for babies under a month of age if they are kissed by someone with an active cold sore.

The nursery school also may be a prime setting for transmission. Little children drool a lot—on their clothes, on their toys, and on each other. That saliva may contain hundreds of thousands of small virions, each capable of spreading herpes to an uninfected playmate.

If you've escaped oral herpes during childhood, you still can pick it up later, especially if you have numerous intimate relationships or if you are engaged in certain occupations where there's frequent contact with oral secretions from strangers. Health care workers in both the medical and dental fields are frequently exposed to the virus.

Two specific situations illustrate the contagious potential of oral herpes. The medical literature documents acquisition of herpes simplex virus type 1 during mouth-to-mouth resuscitation and from wrestling, the latter called herpes gladiatorum. The method of transmission during a life-saving mouth-to-mouth contact is obvious (and certainly worth the risk). But one might question the passage of virus from wrestler to wrestler. They don't kiss, but an infected lip of one wrestler rubbed against a cut or mat burn on the opponent's body may result in a new case of herpes.

Herpes simplex does not survive in air. Transmission requires direct contact with large droplets containing living cells. In other words, you won't catch herpes just by being in the vicinity of a carrier who coughs or sneezes.

One of the most hotly debated medical questions of the day: can herpesviruses survive on inanimate objects like towels, glasses, toys, and lipstick? As a scientist with more than 15 years of experience in both basic research and clinical care, I believe that you rarely if ever catch herpes from anything except the body of another person. I have supervised many technologists who work with the virus in laboratory settings. Not one has been infected during occupational duties!

Nevertheless, I recommend you use only your own towels and drinking glasses, and avoid reusing those of others. I sincerely doubt that you'll catch herpes from a drinking glass. But bacteria and other viruses, such as rhinoviruses (common cold viruses) and enteroviruses (like polio), survive for days on inanimate surfaces, and you certainly could catch them.

Prevalence of herpes simplex type 1 infections varies from community to community. Dr. Martin S. Hirsch, a professor of medicine at Massachussetts General Hospital, reports that only 30 to 50 percent of adults in higher socioeconomic groups have antibodies in their bloodstream against herpes simplex, whereas the rates are 80 to 100 percent in lower socioeconomic groups. By puberty, nearly all members of lower socioeconomic groups have been infected, probably as a result of living in crowded quarters. Most laboratories do not discriminate between herpes type 1 antibody and type 2 antibody. If that were done, 80 to 90 percent of individuals with antibody to herpes simplex would have antibody against herpes type 1. Herpes type 1 infections, you see, are still much more common than those caused by herpes simplex type 2.

Primary Oral Herpes

Our primary, or very first, attack of oral herpes tends to be much more severe than recurrent episodes. The primary infection usually happens during childhood but may not occur until adult life. Blisters develop and quickly pop, leaving raw, painful ulcers. The gums and tongue may be especially tender. Fever, generalized weakness, and foul breath sometimes accompany mouth sores. Blisters may appear around the mouth and on the cheeks. Children may be so uncomfortable that they refuse to eat or drink and need to be hospitalized for several days (like Robert's patient in chapter 2). Adults who practice oral-genital sex may develop a sore throat and tonsillitis similar to a strep infection.

Autoinoculation (spread of disease from one part of the body to another) occurs almost exclusively during a primary herpes attack. Young children frequently put their fingers in their mouth and then rub their eyes, sometimes resulting in herpes infections of the eyes and fingers. Children and adults with eczema are especially at risk. Herpes simplex easily spreads from the lips and face to eczematous areas, producing a generalized skin infection called eczema herpeticum. Patients with this condition require treatment and should be seen by their physician at once.

The Utah Study of Recurrence

About 75 percent of the total U.S. population has antibody circulating in their bloodstream against herpes, reflecting previous infection, and 15 to 30 percent are troubled by recurrences. The most complete analysis of recurrent oral herpes was made by Dr. Spotswood Spruance of the University of Utah. Eighty patients ranging in age from eight to 67 who had experienced frequent cold sores for an average of 18 years were studied. Here are some of his findings:

• Forty-six patients (57 percent) said they averaged a recurrence every one to four months; 19 (24 percent) reported an episode at least every month; and 15 patients (19 percent) said they experienced about two recurrences a year.

• Time from prodrome to eruption of lesions ranged from a few hours in most patients to two days in one person.

• Pain was most intense during the first 24 hours of blistering, declining rapidly thereafter. Less than 10 percent of the patients complained of any pain after six days.

• Clinical recurrences were very short. The blisters would break and crust over within two days with complete healing within eight days, on average.

• Larger blisters required a slightly longer period for healing.

The Trickle Theory of Recurrence

The most widely accepted theory of herpes simplex latency and recurrence was explained in chapter 3. To briefly recount: virus infects

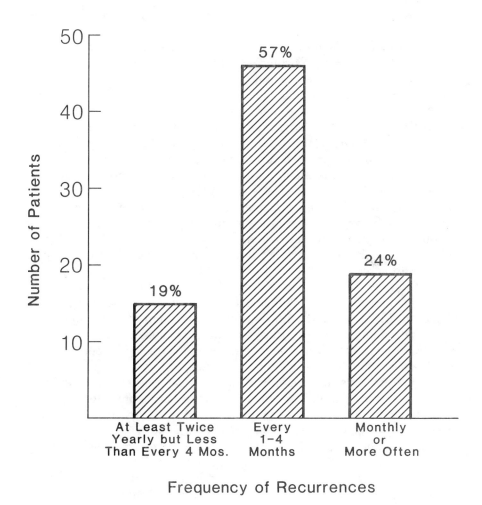

50 ⎤

40

30

20

10

Number of Patients

19%

57%

24%

At Least Twice
Yearly but Less
Than Every 4 Mos.

Every
1–4
Months

Monthly
or
More Often

Frequency of Recurrences

Frequency of recurrences of cold sores among 80 Utah volunteers. Source: S. L.
Spruance et al., "The Natural History of Recurrent Herpes Simplex Labialis: Implications for Antiviral Therapy." *New England Journal of Medicine* 297 (1977):69–75

the body, causes disease, then migrates up nerve pathways to a ganglion, where it hibernates for an indefinite period until reawakened by a stimulus. In genital herpes, virions hibernate in ganglia near the sacral area of our spinal cord. In oral herpes, virions hide in the trigeminal ganglion, located inside our skull near the base of the brain.

But I would like to offer another theory that may provide a better understanding of viral persistence. I call this concept the trickle theory. Think of herpes migrating up and down the nerve pathways like water flowing through a garden hose. The hose is never completely turned off. Instead of becoming inactive, herpes reproduces itself very slowly, and mature new virions leak down the nerve pathway like water dripping from a nozzle. Some water continues to drip out, but you never notice because the droplets are absorbed into the ground. The same thing may happen when the virus trickles down to the skin. Our immune system mops up the few stray particles and prevents a major eruption of cold sores—no puddle, no problem. At the start of an active infection, virions pour down nerve pathways, just as a garden hose sprays a powerful and steady stream when turned on full blast. The viral particles temporarily break through our immune defenses, and we break out in cold sores.

Why does the virus trickle down the nerve instead of flooding the pathways with progeny? Perhaps, through eons of time, herpes has learned to live in concert with its host. Rather than overwhelming the host with billions of viral particles that might cause extensive disease and prove fatal, the virus spawns just enough of itself to permit comfortable survival for both host and parasite.

Some patients, like Doug the landscape architect, claim they can actually feel a pulsation—the effects of the virus trickling. But we have more than anecdotal evidence for this alternative theory. In the absence of any symptoms, some patients carry live virus in their mouths. These patients may be in the trickle phase of the recurrence cycle where so little virus exists that no symptoms surface.

This theory certainly makes sense when you consider the stories of Doug and others who feel continual tingling on their lips. Unless they keep their lips covered with lip ice as a shield against physical provocation, they have almost constant eruptions.

In summary, the trickle theory of recurrence suggests that herpes simplex viruses exist in the host in a dynamic rather than latent state. The tiny virions are always active, but our immune system can keep them in check until a traumatic event—an emotional trigger or physical irritant—upsets the fragile balance between host and parasite, giving the virus the upper hand.

At the University of Minnesota, we're applying the trickle theory to another member of the herpes clan: varicella-zoster virus. We're studying elderly patients who suffer postherpetic neuraglia, the lingering pain associated with shingles. Shingles is caused by varicella-zoster virus. We suspect there might be slow multiplication of the varicella-zoster virus inside the painful nerve all the time. If so, pain might be alleviated if the virus activity could be shut off by an antiviral drug. (More on this in chapter 6).

Sun and Wind Intensify Oral Herpes

Many patients complain that their recurrences of oral herpes follow exposure to the wind and sun while snow skiing, sailing, or beachcombing. Why? Not only are the sun's rays striking your body directly, but they are also being reflected off the snow or water. Wind velocity increases as you ski or sail into the breeze. In other words, you're receiving a bigger dose of the stimulus—much too much for your body to handle. Physical irritation damages our skin slightly. The outside part of the cell, its membrane, develops a small tear due to heat rays from the sun or drying by the wind. Perhaps by creeping through miniscule rents in cell membranes, herpes penetrates weakened cells more efficiently than strong, healthy ones. Certain ultraviolet rays in sunshine actually weaken the immune defenses of our skin cells—another factor facilitating the spread of herpes.

Fever and the Blister

Do cold sores cause fever, or does fever cause cold sores? Recurrent oral herpes is rarely a febrile disease. Fever is the symptom of another infection that's stressing our immune system. The immune defense is called into the field to do battle against a new invading virus, such as influenza. With its legions occupied combating the flu, the immune system cannot protect all borders. Herpes escapes, and we break out in fever blisters (a synonym for cold sores). In other words, the flu engages enough of our immune defenses to make us temporarily immunosuppressed vis-a-vis herpes.

Reinfection

Reinfection means something entirely different than reactivation. Reinfection occurs when a second herpes simplex strain invades your body, whereas reactivation denotes another infection from the same strain already present within your body. There's no doubt you can be reinfected by more than one strain. However, reinfection most likely accounts for a very small percentage of recurrent episodes of oral herpes.

There are increasing hints—scientists call these "soft data"—that a previous infection by herpes simplex type 1 offers some protection against a later infection by type 2 virus. These soft data include the finding that lower socioeconomic groups have a lower incidence of genital herpes. As I've noted, a larger percentage of persons in this group have had herpes type 1 during childhood, a circumstance which may provide protection against acquiring type 2 genital infection later on.

Caring for Cold Sores

• Keep the lesions clean and dry. Occlusive preparations such as petroleum jelly may prolong the attack. Rubbing or biting of the lips or mouth sores exacerbates and possibly lengthens the attack.

• Numbing agents for the lips are available by prescription, but aspirin or acetaminophen-containing preparations may be sufficient for moderate pain and discomfort.

• If sores are present inside the mouth, avoid solid foods until the lesions begin to heal. Compensate by increasing your intake of liquids and soft foods (soup, gelatin).

• Saltwater mouthwashes may help reduce swelling. (Use one teaspoon of table salt per quart of lukewarm water.)

• Stay out of the sun and wind as much as possible.

• Reduce stress. (Tips on stress reduction are found in chapter 3.)

• Don't kiss anyone when your lesions are present. Are there any exceptions? Yes! In a longstanding relationship, you may already have kissed your partner when your cold sores were active. If your partner did not get cold sores then, he or she most likely is immune and kissing need not be curtailed.

• In cases of mouth sores, 2 percent viscous xylocaine applied with a cotton swab directly on the sores may temporarily relieve pain. For this, you will need a prescription.

• Your doctor may prescribe acyclovir ointment. Many patients have told me that if they apply ointment as soon as they feel the prodrome, cold sores don't erupt or run a very mild course. This is very good news for the many victims of oral herpes who dread appearing in public when their herpes is active. The herpes phobia now extends to oral as well as genital disease—one of my technologists told me that during a bout of cold sores, people moved away from her at the lunch counter.

Cold Sores or Canker Sores?

Canker sores are recurrent ulcers that occur only inside the mouth. Although we don't know what causes them, canker sores are not due to herpes and are not contagious. A recent theory suggests that canker sores result from an aberrant immune attack on our own mouth tissues. Canker sores can be quite painful. Temporary relief often follows local application of viscous xylocaine, for which you need a prescription. Your doctor can distinguish canker sores from herpes and other causes of mouth sores on the basis of a physical exam and viral culture, or microscopic examination of cells collected from your mouth.

HERPES IN THE EYE

Dr. Deborah P. Langston, an eye surgeon on the faculty of the Harvard Medical School and an experienced herpes researcher, calls herpes simplex in her book *Living with Herpes* "the most common cause of blindness due to infection in the entire North American continent." But she is quick to point out that herpes eye disease is still relatively uncommon, afflicting approximately one of every 500 people. Fortunately, herpes rarely infects both eyes.

Virus can reach the eyes by direct inoculation. This frequently happens when small children first acquire oral herpes, put their hands in their mouths, and then rub their eyes. Virus also can reach the eye via the left or right trigeminal ganglion. Nerve pathways from these two ganglia lead to the surface of our eyes as well as the lips and mouth. Thus you could acquire cold sores on the lips and later experience a recurrence in the eye.

In children, herpes usually attacks the conjunctiva (a membrane that lines the eyelids and covers the white portions of our eyes), resulting in swelling and redness. Since conjunctivitis has many causes, herpes eye disease in children frequently goes undiagnosed and untreated, but clears spontaneously anyway.

In adults, herpes most often attacks the cornea (outer clear window) of the eye. We refer to this form of eye infection as keratitis. The first symptoms are blurred vision and photophobia (discomfort or intolerance for bright light). Adults with herpes keratitis don't have much redness and usually do not complain of pain, although they sometimes have the sensation that a foreign body is in their eye. Your doctor recognizes herpes keratitis by touching the corner of your eye with a piece of filter paper containing fluorescein and then seeing, under a blue light, the typical pattern of herpes. Herpes lesions of the cornea are called dendrites; they resemble tiny branches of a tree that has lost its leaves. If the dendrites are very small, the doctor may need to use an instrument called a slit lamp to see them. Then the doctor applies a topical anesthetic to numb your cornea and scrapes away the infected cells. Specific antiviral drops or ointment then can be prescribed.

Herpes may not limit itself to the cornea but extend deeper into the eye. If infection spreads to the iris or the eye lens, you feel a deep aching pain. Herpes iritis must be treated because the iris can scar, blocking drainage of the natural fluid formed in the eye. As fluid continues to form, pressure builds up inside the eye, creating a condition called glaucoma. Untreated, glaucoma can eventually lead to blindness. Cataracts may result from recurrent herpetic iritis or from glaucoma.

If you develop "pink eye," blurred vision, or photophobia, please seek medical care. Although uncommon, herpes keratitis is easily recognized on physical examination and confirmed by a simple lab test. A swab specimen from the eye examined under the microscope will reveal the herpes-induced giant cells described earlier in this chapter. I recommend that an ophthalmologist (M.D. eye specialist) be consulted if the diagnosis is herpes. A few patients eventually require surgery to treat cataracts or relieve glaucoma. An ophthalmologist can best judge when surgery is appropriate. If you have herpes keratitis, avoid rubbing the infected eye. Wash your hands if you inadvertently do so. In that way, there is no chance that you will spread herpes to distant parts of your body or to other people.

HERPES OF THE FINGERS (HERPETIC WHITLOWS)

Whitlow, derived from middle English, means a white flaw. Herpetic whitlows are pimplelike sores of the fingers that resemble a whitish abscess if they coalesce. This form of herpes is an occupational hazard for medical and dental personnel who routinely examine patients' mouths. A small cut in the cuticle is sufficient to let herpes in. We theorize that during the first herpes whitlow attack, virus migrates along nerve fibers all the way up the arm, across the shoulder, and into a ganglion near the spinal cord. Recurrences occur when virus migrates through nerve pathways back down the arm to the finger. Whitlows recur less frequently than oral herpes, herpes keratitis, or genital herpes.

Whitlows are often misdiagnosed as bacterial infections. Some patients have even undergone extensive local surgical procedures to drain these whitlows. Patients with herpetic whitlow, particularly for the first time, can be contagious. For example, Robert, the young doctor in chapter 2, bit his nails after examining a pediatric patient with oral herpes. He then inoculated his mouth with his infected finger.

Whitlow is usually caused by herpes type 1, the result of finger-oral contact. However, type 2 whitlows can occur in patients with genital herpes who manipulate their lesions during a primary episode. Therefore, I advise patients with either oral or genital herpes not to touch their lesions when applying medication. A glove or cot should be worn to protect the finger.

Because whitlows are deeper than lip or genital sores, local antiviral therapy at best will only be partially effective. For most patients, whitlows heal within two weeks, and discomfort is minimal. Some patients, however, report severe pain, which limits motion of the involved fingers or even the entire hand. A medical artist who works in our hospital has difficulty drawing for a week to 10 days after a recurrence. If you suffer incapacitating pain or limitation of motion, consult a physician who might consider giving you systemic antiviral drugs.

HERPES ENCEPHALITIS

Encephalitis, commonly known as "sleeping sickness," involves inflammation and swelling of the brain. Because of its insidious onset and potentially severe consequences, the disease frightens patients and baffles doctors. Encephalitis can be fatal, and some survivors are left with permanent brain damage.

There is no single cause of encephalitis. The majority of cases result from a primary viral attack. In the summertime, encephalitis is most commonly due to arboviruses carried by mosquitoes and ticks or enteroviruses spread person-to-person. Mumps was the leading cause of winter or springtime encephalitis before the advent of mumps vaccine. Herpes encephalitis occurs year-round and strikes every age group. Experts' estimates of the number of cases of herpes encephalitis vary from a few hundred to a few thousand in the United States every year.

Herpes encephalitis is not contagious in the typical sense because patient-to-patient spread has never been documented. Exactly how we catch herpes encephalitis remains a mystery. Acquisition of the virus seems to happen asymptomatically: there are no other signs of the disease such as cold sores or eye lesions. Virus apparently enters the nose and progresses from olfactory cells in the nasal passages into a collection of nerve pathways called the olfactory bulb. The virus marches relentlessly toward the brain, where it destroys vital nerve cells. Since herpes type 1 most often infects the nose, lips, and mouth, we would expect herpes encephalitis to be caused by type 1 virus. Indeed that is the case. About 95 percent of all herpes simplex viruses recovered from the brain are type 1.

Herpes encephalitis is *not* a complication of genital herpes. Nor does it often follow reactivation of oral or facial herpes as some publications for the lay public have suggested. Herpes encephalitis is a primary infection in most cases; we have proof of this from antibody testing of patients.

Warning signals are the same for all forms of encephalitis: headache, fever, mild stupor. Later, the patient becomes lethargic, suffers blurred vision, and loses coordination as more of the nervous system becomes involved. Some patients finally fall into a deep coma.

Because the early symptoms are not distinctive, doctors may have difficulty correctly diagnosing encephalitis until infection has spread throughout the brain, killing millions of nerve cells and causing irreparable damage. Brain cells, unlike skin cells, never regenerate. By the time the patient is hospitalized, the disease has often taken an irrevocable toll.

Confirmation of herpes encephalitis requires a brain biopsy—a surgical procedure to remove a small piece of brain tissue after a hole has been drilled through the skull. Only by viewing the herpes under the electron microscope or growing virus from the biopsy specimen can we be sure that the patient suffers from herpes encephalitis and not some other neurologic disorder.

Following are the nearly verbatim excerpts of case reports from medical journals that chronicle the disease in two of my patients:

Case 1

A 22-month-old girl was admitted to the University of Minnesota Hospitals because of seizures and lethargy. The patient was entirely well until three weeks before admission, when she fell out of bed to the floor two feet below, striking her head. The patient did not lose consciousness and appeared normal to the parents after the injury. Eight days before admission, the patient became increasingly drowsy and less responsive. She had seizures that consisted of twitching of the left eyelid, left corner of the mouth, and left upper arm. She was hospitalized elsewhere. When her condition did not improve over the next five days, she was transferred to University of Minnesota Hospitals. Physical examination revealed a lethargic female child in no acute distress. Although the admission diagnosis was viral encephalitis, the history of head trauma made subdural hematoma (bleeding beneath the skull compressing the brain) a strong diagnostic possibility.

Comment: The case of this little girl, whom I'll call Shelly, was reported in the *Journal of Pediatrics* because a brain scan was used to make the diagnosis preoperatively. At surgery, Shelly was found to have herpes encephalitis, not a blood clot. Her case was typical because we never learned how she acquired herpes in the first place, and she experienced a progressive downhill course at first. But unlike most patients with herpes encephalitis, Shelly recovered on her own.

A brain scan involves injecting radioactive material into an arm vein. The substance circulates throughout the body, and if the brain is diseased, radioactivity lingers there awhile. A localized "hot spot" of radioactivity in brain tissue behind the temple bone is most likely herpes encephalitis.

The brain scan has become one of three diagnostic tests for herpes encephalitis. The other two are the electroencephalogram (brain wave test) and the CAT scan. CAT stands for computed axial tomography, an application of computer technology that enhances the ability of X rays to provide a sharp picture of structures inside our body. Although more benign than a biopsy, none of these diagnostic tests is as reliable. The tests are not positive in all cases of the infection; nor are they negative in all cases of noninfection.

Medicine continues to search for an alternative to the brain biopsy. The procedure is invasive and potentially harmful to the patient because the needle may remove healthy tissue as well as herpes-infected cells.

Follow-up: Shelly is 20 years old and attending college, having graduated from high school with honors. Because she was hospitalized in the days before antiviral therapy, her case illustrates the strange, inscrutable behavior of herpesviruses in some hosts who are able to defeat the virus by themselves.

Case 2

A 17-month-old girl was admitted to the University of Minnesota Hospitals because of seizures and right-sided paralysis. At age two months a "white film" had been noted over the left eye. On the basis of a dendritic ulcer, an ophthalmologist made the clinical diagnosis of herpes keratitis and began treatment with idoxuridine drops. The herpes keratitis cleared, but glaucoma developed, necessitating surgery.

Nine days before she was admitted, her parents had noted increasing lethargy. That evening she had her first seizure, with her head and eyes turning to the right and shaking of the right side, followed by a generalized convulsion. On neurological examination, she responded neither to her name nor to a loud noise. Deep pain was perceived in all four extremities, but she did not cry. There was no blink response to threatening motion, although occasionally she appeared to follow objects. A craniotomy was performed the same day. The brain, which was under great tension without pulsation, was softened, and the left temporal lobe was necrotic (composed of dead tissue). A left temporal biopsy was taken for histology and cultures.

On the fifth hospital day, Herpesvirus hominis encephalitis was confirmed, and on the sixth hospital day treatment with cytarabine was begun. The clinical deterioration was arrested temporarily, but on the eighteenth hospital day, fever and seizures recurred. Two subsequent courses of cytarabine were given. Fever slowly subsided over a period of several weeks. The seizures remained a problem, and the child required administration of multiple anticonvulsants.

She was discharged after three months of hospitalization, with a residual right hemiplegia (paralysis of the right side of the body), language loss, seizure disorder, and apparent mental retardation.

Comment: The case of this child, whom I'll call Carrie, was unusual because we were able to confirm a previous herpes infection in the eye. Carrie was the exception, rather than the rule: most patients with herpes encephalitis do not have lesions anywhere except the brain. Unfortunately for Carrie, the antiviral therapy she received was later proven ineffective, and the little girl experienced some sequelae (residual problems). Effective therapies now are being developed. The antiviral drug vidarabine has been slow to significantly reduce the mortality of this condition. (For more information on therapy, see chapter 9.)

Diagnosing and treating herpes encephalitis presents medical science with a major challenge. Dr. Richard Whitley, who heads a national research team studying treatment of herpes encephalitis, wrote in the January 15, 1982, issue of the *Journal of the American Medical Association*:

Herpes simplex encephalitis defies clinical and diagnostic definition by routine procedures. At best, physician judgment will be correct only three of four times, a frequency too low to suggest that patients with suspected cases be treated with potentially toxic drugs without an established diagnosis. . . . It is hoped that with the development of newer diagnostic methods, noninvasive procedures will be developed to avoid the need for routine brain biopsy in the future.

HERPES AND WEAKENED IMMUNITY

Since the dawn of organ transplantation in the mid-1960s, surgeons and immunologists have been playing a tricky and sometimes precarious game with mother nature. They have learned to "fool" the body into believing the transplanted kidney, heart, liver, pancreas, or bone marrow is part of its own biological makeup.

The body's natural response is to launch an immunological arsenal against all invaders, rejecting both friendly (such as the donor organ) and unfriendly (such as bacteria or viruses) guests.

Scientists subvert the body's rejection system by tissue typing—finding a close match from a relative or cadaver—and by immunosuppressive therapy, the use of drugs that weaken the immune response. Immunosuppressive therapy is a two-edged sword: by enhancing the chances of keeping the new organ, we make the patient vulnerable to infection. Cancer patients also sustain immunosuppression during chemotherapy. As the cancer-fighting agents rid the body of destructive mutant cells, they also eliminate healthy, disease-fighting cells, leaving the patients susceptible to infection because the delicate balance between host and parasite has been tipped in favor of the bugs.

The University of Minnesota helped pioneer transplant surgery and, likewise, the science of immunology. The world's first pancreas transplant was performed here in 1966; the first bone marrow transplant in 1968; potent antirejection medicine called antilymphocyte globulin was developed here, also in 1968; and the first mobile system for preservation of transplantable organs established in 1970. Today Minnesota operates the busiest pediatric transplant program in the world and is one of the few places that will accept diabetics for kidney transplantation.

As doctors monitor a transplant patient's recovery, they watch closely for any signs of rejection and infection. If unchecked, even a simple infection can result in a serious threat to the patient and possible rejection of the organ. About two-thirds of all transplant patients experience some form of postoperative viral infection. Because most of these infections are due to herpesviruses, Minnesota naturally became a major center for development of antiviral drugs against the herpes family.

Patients with a history of cold sores will almost certainly have recurrences after transplant. Even patients who've never had a cold sore are likely to break out with oral herpes because the vast majority of us have the virus dormant in our nerve cells. In transplant patients, blisters often cover the inside of the mouth, and may extend into the esophagus, causing pain on swallowing and difficulty eating. Herpes even may invade the lungs to cause pneumonia or the liver to produce hepatitis without revealing its presence in the mouth or on the skin. Such was the case with an 11-month-old Massachussetts girl, whose story is a dramatic example of the successful marriage of surgical innovation and modern immunology. On the brink of a historic victory over liver failure, this child was imperiled by the commonplace herpes simplex virus.

Jamie Fiske and Herpes Hepatitis

In 1982, Jamie Fiske sparked renewed interest in organ transplantation when she underwent a life-saving liver transplant that drew national attention, largely because of her father's unprecedented appeal for an organ made before a national convention of the American Academy of Pediatrics in New York City.

Jamie was most susceptible to infection in the first few weeks after surgery when she received high doses of the antirejection medication cyclosporine. Therefore, it was not surprising that about two weeks after transplant, Jamie developed a high fever—usually the first signal of infection or rejection—and then pneumonia. Jamie's father, Charles, recalls: "It was an emotional time for us because Jamie had just been removed from the respirator and we felt we had passed a major milestone; it seemed that with every step forward there were 10 steps backward. I remember Dr. [Nancy] Ascher [assistant professor of surgery] saying that she would rather have it be rejection than herpes because they could control the rejection while they weren't sure they could control the infection."

After three days of a worrisome elevated temperature, at one point topping 102 degrees Fahrenheit, a biopsy of the new liver was ordered. Results showed that Jamie's liver was not being rejected, but strange cells indicating herpes infection were discovered. Doctors recorded their impression: herpes simplex infection of the lungs and liver.

One month earlier, the federal Food and Drug Administration had approved intravenous use of the new antiherpes drug called acyclovir. One of the key drug-testing centers had been the University of Minnesota. After consultation with our Clinical Virology Service, the transplanters placed Jamie on acyclovir.

There were some tense moments for the family and medical staff alike as they waited to see if acyclovir would arrest the spreading infection. The viral attack certainly had the potential of growing into a serious—even fatal—problem. But doctors remained optimistic, partly because of acyclovir's success in treating other herpes infections in transplant patients at our medical center. Jamie's parents endured this ordeal as they had others—confident their daughter would rally.

Chief surgeon John Najarian would later call her response "remarkable." Within three days, Jamie's fever began to fall, and her course of recovery was back on schedule. If the infection had continued to spread unchecked, Jamie's new liver could have been lost.

As a postscript, her father told us that Jamie experienced an outbreak of fever blisters about 11 months after surgery—not surprising in view of the earlier herpes infection.

CONCLUSION: HERPES "COMPLEX"

The story of Jamie Fiske illustrates that the marvelous advances of modern organ transplantation can be threatened by the usually trivial but ubiquitous herpes simplex. Herpes complicates the hospital course of complex immunosuppressed patients. Herpes type 1 is also responsible for cold sores, the most common herpes disease in the general population. We have covered the spectrum of herpes simplex infections involving the mouth, lips, eyes, fingers, and brain. As we've learned, the varied and intriguing ways that herpes simplex interacts with our bodies are not simple at all. Perhaps herpes simplex should be renamed herpes complex.

Chickenpox: Mild for Most, Devastating for Others

Sick children bring physicians face to face with their own mortality. They force you to question the power of medicine and your abilities as a doctor. At times, they make you feel impotent because medical science can be fallible. Yet a suffering child, like no other patient, challenges and inspires you to find better ways to treat disease and cope with pain.

Michael Peterson was that kind of youngster. He remains one of my most memorable patients.

MIKE'S FIGHT FOR LIFE

I can still recall with vivid detail our first meeting. It was in the emergency room of University of Minnesota Hospitals just a few years ago. He was 10, with curly blonde hair and a bubbling laugh. Nurses were wrapping his arm for a blood pressure check when I entered the ward. He was obviously nervous; his anxiety surfaced in the form of nonstop chatter about a Florida vacation that unexpectedly was cut short.

His mother, Patricia, in her early thirties, sat near the examining table, awaiting word on her son. After a brief examination of Mike, I turned to counsel Mrs. Peterson. She was overwhelmed with emotion. "Please help Mike," she pleaded.

Eighteen months earlier, Mike had developed acute lymphoblastic leukemia, a cancer that attacks the body's white blood cells. As explained in chapter 1, white cells form the backbone of the body's infection-fighting immune system. Lymphocytes, one type of white cell, play a key role in the immune defense by recognizing and remembering foreign invaders such as viruses. In Mike's type of leukemia, the lymphocytes are abnormal, and the immune system, as a result, is suppressed. Such immunosuppressed patients are highly susceptible to many infections, especially chickenpox.

Thanks to early diagnosis and powerful anticancer drugs, Mike's leukemia was put into remission. All visible signs of the disease disappeared. He missed only a few weeks of school.

Despite successful induction of remission with chemotherapy, doctors cautioned Mike's parents that his leukemia could recur. Scientists still are unable to explain why some individuals are permanently cured of cancer and others suffer relapses.

But we are sure of one thing: any child who is immunosuppressed and exposed to chickenpox, caused by varicella-zoster virus, runs a risk of developing a life-threatening infection. The patient may be cured of cancer only to die from a usually trivial childhood illness. Unfortunately, Michael Peterson was the unusual child with cancer who had escaped chickenpox until age 10.

The Exposure

Every Minnesotan complains about the seemingly endless winters. Survival takes many forms: some capitalize on their cold environment and become involved in outdoor activities. Others opt for winter vacations in warmer climes. This winter was particularly long and cold with subfreezing temperatures extending into March. The airlines enjoyed a banner year as Minnesotans flocked to Florida in record numbers.

Like many of their friends and neighbors, the Peterson family decided to spend a week in Florida. They accepted an invitation from Pat's sister, Debbie Johnson, who lived near Tampa Bay. It was not an easy decision for the Petersons. Although Mike seemed to have totally recovered from his cancer, there was a lingering apprehension that the disease would reappear. Anything out of the ordinary, even an airplane trip, was fraught with some anxiety for the family because doctors don't know what brings on leukemia or triggers a relapse. Nevertheless, the thought of a week of sunny days was too compelling. At the last minute, Mike's father was forced to stay in Minneapolis because of business commitments. So mother and son were off to Florida.

The flight south was uneventful. Thrilled by his very first plane ride, Mike babbled about geography, jet engines, and a visit to Disney World. As the plane landed, however, Pat noticed that her ears were somewhat uncomfortable and her nose felt a little stuffy. She attributed her discomfort to the change in cabin pressure. But Pat's stuffy head worsened through the evening, forcing her to bed early. Because her sister's home was a small three-bedroom rambler and she had children of her own, Pat and Mike stayed in the den, sharing a rollabed couch. As Pat undressed, she noticed some pimplelike spots on her neck. She could almost imagine that they itched. Tired, she shrugged her shoulders, put on her nightgown, and went to bed.

When she awoke the next morning, Pat felt feverish. She looked in the mirror and discovered that the spots on her neck had become little blisters. Many other red spots appeared on her face and chest. She turned and saw that her back was also covered.

Trying to control her panic, Pat called her sister into the bathroom for advice. Debbie, a schoolteacher, recognized the problem at once. She had seen that rash many times in her fifth grade classroom. "Pat, you have chickenpox. What a gas!" she exclaimed.

Debbie recalled that Pat was the only sibling in the family who had escaped chickenpox as a child. Pat was in Washington, D.C., for a week on a class field trip when her sister and brother experienced the viral attack. "But adults can't get chickenpox, can they?" Pat wondered. She finally accepted the diagnosis after calling the Johnson's pediatrician, who warned Pat that chickenpox in adults can lead to pneumonia.

With the chickenpox confirmed, Pat was convinced that she must return to Minneapolis as quickly as possible because of Mike. Her sister pleaded with her to seek medical help at a nearby hospital.

Pat rejected that idea, saying, "Deb, when the doctors at the University first explained all the problems with acute leukemia, they told me that if Mike were ever exposed to chickenpox he must go to University Hospitals at once for a special transfusion. Mike has never had chickenpox, and if he comes down with it now it could be very, very serious."

Mother and son faced a series of frustrations in trying to get home. It was Sunday, and only a few flights were available. They finally obtained a booking on the next-to-last flight to Minneapolis. As they were boarding their plane, a flight attendant asked Pat if she could explain the rash on her face. When Pat mentioned chickenpox, the flight attendant conferred with several other airline personnel. This led to a discussion among the airport authorities. Pat and Mike were bumped from their flight and detained for several hours before the local health officials advised the airline that the Petersons could return to Minneapolis without jeopardizing other passengers. They barely made the last northbound flight.

Mike and his mother arrived in Minneapolis late Sunday evening. They rushed from the airport to University of Minnesota Hospitals. The oncologist (cancer specialist) who treated Mike's leukemia asked that I be available to examine the boy when he arrived. It was the first time that I had met the Petersons.

Mrs. Peterson's appearance relieved me at once. The chickenpox rash was mild, her color good, and her breathing normal. She was obviously experiencing a typical chickenpox infection. The rash would last a total of five days, heal without scarring, and leave her completely unscathed. We advised Mrs. Peterson that the outcome for Mike, unfortunately, might be different. We therefore would have to embark on an attempt to prevent him from contracting the disease.

Trying to Prevent Chickenpox

The only way to protect pox-vulnerable children like Mike Peterson is to reinforce their immune system. We do this by giving them plasma or globulin from others who have antibodies to the chickenpox virus. In a sense, we are borrowing a part of the healthy immune system from someone else.

In 1972, the Clinical Virology Service at the University of Minnesota, in conjunction with the Hospital Blood Bank, launched a program to collect blood plasma from individuals who had experienced recent episodes of shingles. When a person is sick, the body normally makes disease-fighting antibodies. These antibodies attack the specific virus causing one's illness. Antibodies in the bloodstream of patients recovering from shingles (also known as zoster) will protect anyone exposed to chickenpox because the same virus causes both chickenpox and shingles. We call the antibody-containing material ZIP, an acronym for zoster immune plasma.

Before the start of the ZIP Program, most immunosuppressed children who were closely exposed suffered a chickenpox attack. Without a medical attempt to prevent infection, called prophylaxis, one of every 10 childhood leukemia patients with chickenpox died. ZIP, however, can only prevent infection; it can't be used to treat the illness once the pox emerge.

We gave Mike ZIP intravenously and observed him afterward for an allergic reaction that sometimes follows transfusion of foreign plasma. No problems arose, and Mike was sent home the same night. Everything seemed to be going well for exactly two weeks. Then, to our dismay, the boy broke out in chickenpox. The mother telephoned us several times a day. From her reports, the viral illness apparently was following a normal course: first a fever and next the rash. There was nothing extraordinary about the viral attack for the first two days. Then Mike began to complain of weakness and had some difficulty breathing. His rash was spreading rapidly. We thought the wisest course was to hospitalize the boy. To protect other children on the same ward, we placed Mike in strict isolation—in a separate room where all who entered were required to wear gown, mask, and gloves.

For three days Mike appeared to be holding his own. On the fourth hospital day his lungs began to weaken. A chest X ray confirmed our suspicions—Mike had chickenpox pneumonia. Each day Mike became a little sicker, his breathing more labored and rapid. By the seventh day Mike obviously was losing ground. New lesions were continuing to spread over his body. He stopped drinking and had to be fed through an intravenous tube. His breathing was irregular; his vital signs were unstable. During the night he was placed on a respirator because his lungs were unable to exchange gases effectively. His chickenpox was out of control!

Based on my past experience, I knew that when children required this type of extreme supportive therapy for chickenpox, they usually did not survive. The medical team decided the time had come to discuss the inevitable with mother and father. The session was heart-wrenching for everyone.

Finally, on the eighth day of hospitalization, Mike lapsed into a coma. He died with his parents at his bedside.

Mike's death was especially traumatic for the family because he was the Petersons' only child. His mother felt tremendous guilt for she had exposed Mike to chickenpox. We assured her that she had done all she could to save her little boy. She had notified us as soon as possible of the chickenpox exposure. Everything else was in the province of medicine and nature. Why had ZIP failed? Most likely because Mike experienced an intimate exposure. In other words, he received far too much virus for the transfused antibodies to neutralize. The circumstances of the Florida trip put Mike in very close contact with his mother when she was most contagious.

The medical team also agonized over Michael's death. He represented the first failure of ZIP in a long time. We wondered if our dosage calculations had been wrong, or if the plasma was too old to be effective. In the final analysis, this was a sad example of the fallibility of trying to prevent viral infections using someone else's antibodies. It doesn't always work.

Mike—an Exceptional Case

Most children are not going to die from chickenpox, nor are they likely to suffer any serious complications. Yet the story of Mike illustrates the potentially devastating effects of this normally mild childhood illness. His case emphasizes the absolute necessity of seeking medical help for immunosuppressed youngsters as soon as possible after any type of chickenpox exposure.

If Mike contracted chickenpox today, he might still be alive. Drugs have been developed to treat the virus, giving immunosuppressed patients who develop chickenpox despite prophylaxis at least a fighting chance.

THE TYPICAL CHICKENPOX STORY

Chickenpox is the most common rash disease of childhood. About 98 percent of us will experience chickenpox by the age of 18. Rubella and measles have virtually disappeared, thanks to effective vaccines, but a similar means of preventing chickenpox is not yet generally available.

Though chickenpox is much less contagious than measles, we estimate that if it is introduced into a household, more than half of the susceptible members will become infected. You usually catch chickenpox through close contact with a carrier. Chickenpox can easily spread through elementary schools and day care centers, probably a result of breathing air contaminated by infected classmates.

Chickenpox is seasonal, with upsurges beginning in late winter, peaking in April or May. Chickenpox can occur in any month of the year, but cases are uncommon during the summer and early fall.

The typical incubation period is 14 to 16 days, but can be as short as 11 days or as long as three weeks. Rash first breaks out on the chest and back, then spreads to the face, scalp, arms, and legs. The rash at first appears to be slightly raised bumps (papules). Papules fill with fluid—often within hours after erupting—to become vesicles. The presence of tiny thin-roofed vesicles indicates the virus is active, multiplying rapidly in the body. Vesicles can erupt virtually anywhere—even inside the mouth, nose, and ears. The vesicular fluid turns cloudy by the third or fourth day as white cells come into the area to fight infection. The vesicles are then called pustules, meaning blisters containing pus. Pustules normally become scabs in five to six days. The scabs fall off in 10 to 14 days, almost invariably leaving no scar.

HOW THE VIRUS MAKES YOU SICK

Most diseases caused by the herpes family require direct contact for their spread, usually kissing or sexual activity. Chickenpox is an exception. Patients with chickenpox shed virus in their respiratory secretions and from their rash. Therefore, chickenpox spreads through the air as well as by direct contact with the vesicles. The virus does not survive very long outside the human body. To catch chickenpox you must be close to someone who has the illness, probably within a few inches.

As you breathe in air containing varicella-zoster virus, hundreds of thousands of tiny virions impact against the cells lining your nasal passages. Each virion can penetrate the main portion of your cell, called the cytoplasm. There the virus literally undresses, taking itself apart. The hereditary unit of the virus, double-stranded DNA, migrates from the cytoplasm into your cell's nucleus. The viral DNA jams the messages normally transmitted by your cell nucleus and begins to send out its own. Your cell now has become a factory manufacturing new viruses. Viral parts are synthesized in the cytoplasm and conveyed to the nucleus, where they are all put together. When nearly complete, the new viral particle leaves the nucleus, clothing itself with a piece of the outside of the nucleus, called the nuclear membrane. New viral particles escape the cell by creeping through its outermost membrane or, in some instances, by actually blowing the cell up. Once outside the cell, they are free to wander on, attach to other cells, and start multiplying all over again.

This entire process of viral assemblage takes several days to a week for the virus to be shed, or become a unit outside the cell. During this period you don't experience any symptoms because very little virus exists in your body. Scientists believe that symptoms, such as fever, are not just the result of the infection but are also part of the body's immune response to the viral invasion. We don't feel sick while the virus is still building itself up inside cells, preparing to launch forays of destruction.

Breaking out of the cell, the virions can go virtually anywhere in the body. Virions move into the little vessels that circulate lymph fluid. These vessels carry virus particles to lymph glands. From lymph glands, varicella-zoster virus may get into the blood. Once in the bloodstream, virions preferentially go to certain organs like the liver and lungs. Again they attach, penetrate the normal cells, and begin to multiply. Another cycle of time—perhaps a week—is required for the virus to multiply in the distant organs. You still feel no symptoms at this point.

At the end of the incubation period, usually two weeks, millions of mature viral particles are released from many sites. Virions infect the blood again, circulate throughout the body, and erupt into the bottom layer of skin cells to cause blisters. You become sick with chills, fever, and weakness as your immune system battles the unwelcome visitors.

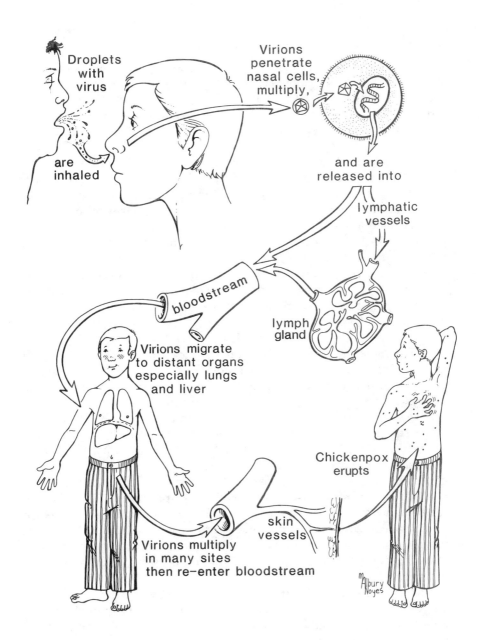

Path of the chickenpox virus.

In addition to carrying the virus to the skin tissue, the blood transports the virus to vital organs of the body. Varicella-zoster virus actually causes vesicles inside our bodies. Minute pockets of disease can be found in the lungs and liver. If you examine gut tissue lining the gastrointestinal tract, you will find small ulcers that developed from broken vesicles.

Almost all of us are strong enough to ward off serious damage. Our immune system surveys the invading foreigners and responds with appropriate reactions to defend us. Our body coats the active virions with neutralizing antibodies, rendering them harmless and preventing any permanent organ destruction. Interferon is produced, a protein that protects cells from further viral incursion. After a few days to a week, the viral attack is repelled.

But, as our chickenpox rash fades, virions silently settle into nerve ganglia up and down our spine. Varicella-zoster virus then hibernates for many years. If the virus wakens, we break out in shingles.

TIPS ON CARE

The most bothersome symptom of chickenpox is the intense itching, driving children to scratch themselves continuously. Scratching may lead to bacterial infection of the pox, resulting in scarring. Some people, especially blacks, have skin that is prone to form scar tissue after the slightest injury—even scratching. How do you prevent scarring? Don't scratch! That may be difficult to control with a youngster. So I suggest keeping fingernails short and clean. Oatmeal baths offer the best relief from severe itching. Be sure to cover your bathtub drain with gauze; the pipes won't find oatmeal appetizing! Cold compresses applied to the itchiest spots may provide symptomatic relief. I do not recommend aspirin for children with chickenpox because the medication has been associated with Reye syndrome. If your child has a high fever, your druggist can provide you with one of many compounds containing acetaminophen, a substance that reduces fever but is unrelated to aspirin.

Two drugs have been shown to be effective in the treatment of chickenpox—acyclovir and vidarabine (more about these in chapter 9). I recommend that all immunosuppressed patients with chickenpox, both adults and children, receive antiviral therapy. Hospitalization usually is necessary because the drugs currently available must be given intravenously in order to be effective. Also, any adult or child with a potentially serious case of chickenpox might benefit from care in a hospital setting. An oral form of acyclovir is now being tested. Should acyclovir capsules prove effective, doctors may offer outpatient care to chickenpox sufferers.

POSSIBLE COMPLICATIONS FOR VARIOUS GROUPS

For most people, chickenpox is a mild disease, causing nothing more than itching and a slight fever. But varicella-zoster virus, like its cousins, is not totally benign. Complications can occur, and the disease proves fatal in about two per 100,000 cases.

Children

The reason I, as a pediatrician, favor chickenpox vaccination for all children—once the appropriate safety and efficacy testing are completed—is that "normal" children do not go entirely scot-free from chickenpox.

A few children develop chickenpox arthritis. The virus actually

---

CHICKENPOX FACT SHEET

Cause: Varicella-zoster virus

Who gets chickenpox: Virtually everyone; 98 percent of the U.S. population contracts chickenpox during childhood

Incubation period: 11 to 21 days, most commonly 14 to 16 days

Who is at risk for complications: Adults; patients with depressed immunity especially those with cancer or organ transplants; infants whose mothers get chickenpox near the time of delivery

Prevention: Injection of chickenpox antibodies as soon as possible after exposure

Tips on care: Oatmeal baths, cold compresses on itchiest spots; short, clean fingernails to prevent bacterial infection of rash; don't use aspirin

Call your doctor if: Fever (>101° F orally) lasts for more than 2 days; new blisters are still forming after 5 days; there is difficulty in walking, talking, or staying awake; breathing is rapid or labored; vomiting develops

---

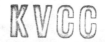

invades the joint, resulting in limitation of movement and discomfort to its victims. Fortunately, the arthritis is temporary.

Chickenpox of the skin causes superficial damage, but in some children the sores can become infected and scar. Chickenpox involving the brain—either by direct extension of the virus or through an exaggerated reaction of the immune system—occurs about once in 2,000 cases. These youngsters may be recovering nicely from the rash and then develop encephalitis, resulting in walking difficulties or decreased state of consciousness. Almost all patients with chickenpox of the nervous system recover without permanent damage.

In 1963, an Australian pathologist, Dr. R. D. K. Reye, and his colleagues described a strange disease that damages the liver and brain. The cause of this condition, called Reye syndrome, is unknown, but the sequence of events has been well described. Children, almost always under the age of 18, contract a viral illness. They appear to be on the road to recovery when vomiting, diarrhea, and disorientation develop suddenly. The patients require hospitalization, and 25 percent of them die despite intensive care. Both influenza B and chickenpox may precede Reye syndrome. Dr. Stephen Preblud of the CDC calculates that Reye syndrome occurs in 3.2 per 100,000 cases of chickenpox.

Adults

The few who escape chickenpox in childhood may have trouble if they contract the disease as adults. We don't understand why, because adults have just as good immune function as children. But in the case of chickenpox something goes awry. One to two percent of adult patients wind up with chickenpox pneumonia requiring a physician's care.

Many adults don't remember their chickenpox. If neither you nor a family member recalls your illness, your doctor can have your blood checked for antibody against varicella-zoster virus. The presence of antibody indicates that you're immune to chickenpox.

Immunosuppressed Patients

A weakened immune system increases the risk of chickenpox complications. Adults or children taking any form of immunosuppressive drugs, including steroids, should be under a physician's care if they develop chickenpox.

Chickenpox rarely occurs a second time in normal individuals. Second attacks tend to be quite mild. Recently I learned that several immunosuppressed adults who had chickenpox as children developed a second case of chickenpoxlike disease after being exposed. If you're immunosuppressed, avoid close contact with a case of chickenpox until medical science sorts out whether or not you truly are susceptible to chickenpox a second time.

Pregnant Women and Infants

A pregnant woman and her newborn child are in danger if she contracts chickenpox. Although rare, chickenpox during pregnancy may damage the baby before birth or cause a serious infection in the infant right after delivery. If a susceptible woman is exposed at any time during pregnancy, she should receive plasma or globulin to prevent chickenpox.

What if the mother develops chickenpox near the time of delivery? In that case, her baby will not be damaged before birth but may sustain a serious infection as a newborn. We allow the delivery to take its normal course. Then we give the baby an injection of varicella-zoster virus antibodies. If chickenpox occurs within the first four weeks of life, we usually admit the baby to the hospital and administer an antiviral drug. Babies cope quite well with chickenpox after one month of age.

Infants exposed to mothers with chickenpox face a special situation. The newborn's immune system is immature, rendering the baby especially prone to infection that can spread uncontrollably. If the mother contracts chickenpox during the last week of pregnancy or the first week after delivery, her baby has a 25 percent chance of developing the disease. The baby may be born with chickenpox because the virus contained in the mother's blood crossed the placenta into the baby's circulation before birth. Or the infant may develop chickenpox after delivery, having been infected by touching the mother's rash or from droplets exhaled by the mother during close contact with her infant.

If you've had childhood chickenpox, is your baby susceptible during the first few months of life? Usually not, because the baby has received antibodies from you during gestation. These antibodies are protective for about six months, unless your baby sustains a very intimate exposure.

One of the questions most frequently asked of me as a pediatrician is: can I take my baby home if there is chickenpox in my household? Yes you may, but keep the baby away from children who have chickenpox or may be incubating the disease. If chickenpox is in the community, any pox-vulnerable child could be harboring the virus. Fondling or kissing transmits a lot of virions. Your infant should not come into direct contact with siblings and other children who may be incubating chickenpox until the baby is at least one month old.

PREVENTION

In the early 1970s, the nation faced a severe shortage of ZIP. Blood banks could not provide prophylaxis for all exposed susceptible children with depressed immunity. Because our medical center specializes in cancer treatment and organ transplantation, we care for many more immunosuppressed children than most hospitals do. Therefore, our needs for ZIP are significantly greater. I recall many instances when I would request ZIP from the blood bank, only to find that their stores were empty. It was terribly frustrating for me as a physician and life-threatening to our patients.

How do you find the necessary plasma when only a few individuals in the community have the correct antibodies in their blood? Since chickenpox and shingles are not reportable diseases to the health department, there is no record of their incidence nor any account of who might help save this particular life.

In 1974, a young girl being treated for cancer at University of Minnesota Hospitals sustained an intimate chickenpox exposure. Because her blood type was unusual, we faced an urgent dilemma—finding the right match. We knew that someone, somewhere in the community, could help the girl. How could we find this anonymous individual with the right blood type to give plasma? We appealed to the public through the news media.

The local press was a useful and cooperative ally. Donations poured in. We received enough plasma to save the little girl and help other immunosuppressed youngsters. Several media appeals in the 1970s provided an ample supply of plasma for future use. The following news account was typical of our media appeals for help:

WANTED: *blood donors, age 17–66, who have suffered from the painful rash of shingles within the past month. The ZIP in their blood may save the lives of some youngsters who otherwise could die from chickenpox. (Minneapolis Tribune, June 4, 1979)*

We have since learned that you don't need shingles patients as donors. Plasma or globulin can be prepared from normal donors with high titers of chickenpox antibody. This material is now available nationally, obviating our need for media appeals.

Antibodies are most effective when given within three days of the exposure. Even then, the postexposure prophylaxis approach is not successful in every patient. About 25 percent of the children still break out in chickenpox, although the disease is usually modified. But in extreme situations, such as Mike's case, patients may develop a life-threatening disease. Therefore, a better method to prevent chickenpox is desperately needed.

Research has turned in recent years toward development of a vaccine. Most viral vaccines in use today are prepared from live virus. Virions are manipulated in the laboratory until they lose their ability to produce disease but still stimulate the immune system. This process of vaccine development, called attenuation, has been successful in the production of measles, rubella, and polio vaccines.

The Japanese have taken the lead in the development of live, attenuated chickenpox vaccine. A group headed by Dr. Michiaki Takahashi of Osaka University reported in 1974 in the international medical journal *Lancet* that chickenpox vaccine was successful in preventing spread of the disease on a children's cancer ward. Since that time, vaccine experiments have moved forward in both Japan and the United States. Children with leukemia in remission are being given a vaccine strain derived from this Japanese discovery to learn if it can protect them from chickenpox. Of course, the most important use of the vaccine would be to protect them during the time they are not in remission. Even though the vaccine has been attenuated, it may not be safe enough for children who are heavily immunosuppressed. Therefore, trials of this vaccine are advancing cautiously.

A major concern hampering the progress of chickenpox vaccine is the problem of latency. Latent virus may later reactivate to cause shingles. Although vaccine development has proceeded slowly, I predict that it is just a matter of time before chickenpox vaccine is available for safe immunization of all normal children.

REFLECTIONS ON A CHILDHOOD DISEASE

Michael Peterson died of chickenpox at the age of 10. His was a rare and unusual case; almost everyone recovers uneventfully and may forget they ever had chickenpox. But Mike's story is unsettling and causes us to reflect. What a curious circumstance that the mildest of all childhood diseases could be fatal if our immune system fails. Herpesviruses are sinister: all of them are potentially devastating for anyone whose immune system is weakened. And even if our immune system stays completely intact, we never totally lose the varicella-zoster virus. The virus survives like seeds of fire in a bed of coals. Sometimes these viral seeds burst into flame as the burning rash of shingles!

Shingles: Seeds of Fire

Like most shingles sufferers, I have tried every means available in modern medicine to combat these painful and sometimes embarrassing outbreaks. —a Wilmington, Delaware, woman

My doctor didn't give me much information about shingles except to say they last a long time. —a Lexington, Kentucky, man

My father-in-law is in his seventies, and has had herpes zoster for 10 years now. It has affected one side of his face and head. He has seen 11 different doctors but to no avail. —a National City, California, woman

I have seen my husband change from a happy man into someone I hardly know any more. —a Helen Springs, Arkansas, woman

These are the voices of people suffering—directly and indirectly—the pain and trauma of shingles, a disease known medically as herpes zoster but sometimes referred to in newspaper stories as the "agony of the aged" or "herpedemic of the elderly." Comments throughout this chapter come from patients, their relatives, and doctors who contacted me at the University of Minnesota following news reports about our shingles research. Extensive press attention was focused on a June 16, 1983, article in the *New England Journal of Medicine* that summarized a two-year shingles study at our university and 19 other medical centers in the United States and Canada. Headlines, such as "Herpes Drug Prevents the Spread of Shingles" in the national newspaper *USA Today*, prompted many to seek detailed information and possible treatment at our hospital.

We received more than 300 letters and telephone calls from across the United States during the following months. The inquirers were confused, frightened, desperate—yet hopeful. Most either were in terrible pain or knew someone who was. The avalanche of correspondence was convincing proof that shingles is a silent epidemic, worthy of the same attention devoted to genital herpes.

How many people suffer from shingles? We can only estimate because there is no official monitoring of the incidence. A retrospective survey of residents from Rochester, Minnesota, identified 590 new cases of shingles during a 15-year period. Adjusting for age based on the 1980 U.S. census, we estimate there are at least 300,000 new cases in the United States each year.

Like other diseases caused by herpesviruses, shingles has been around for centuries. But shingles is unusual because it primarily strikes the elderly, without apparent reason. If you live to be 80 years old you will have a 25 percent chance of a shingles attack. Shingles is a disease that you are likely to hear more about in years to come as the average age of our population increases.

What exactly is shingles? The disease is caused by varicella-zoster virus—the same herpesvirus that's responsible for chickenpox during childhood. Shingles is actually a recurrence of chickenpox, although the two diseases do not look alike. After years of hibernation inside our body, the virions, like seeds of fire, sometimes ignite, causing a burning rash.

The word *shingles* is derived from the Latin *cingulum* meaning *belt* or *girdle*—an appropriate description since the rash appears in girdlelike swaths on the body. *Zoster* is the Greek word for the belt worn by men in ancient Greece. The word apparently was applied to shingles because of the rash's beltlike appearance.

Shingles is rarely life threatening, but I know of two patients whose illness drove them to suicide. Many more patients have threatened to take their own lives.

Shingles is not very well understood, even by some physicians. A young colleague of mine said recently, "When I first read about shingles in medical school, I thought it was a joke," indicating his ignorance about the seriousness of the disorder.

Shingles shares many of the characteristics of diseases caused by the herpes simplex viruses: prodromal symptoms, pain, and a similar course of rash. The viruses even look alike under the electron microscope. But varicella-zoster and herpes simplex viruses behave very differently in the human body, and shingles is in no way related to sexual activity.

The medical term for shingles, herpes zoster, has confused many people and even embarrassed some shingles sufferers. I know a maid

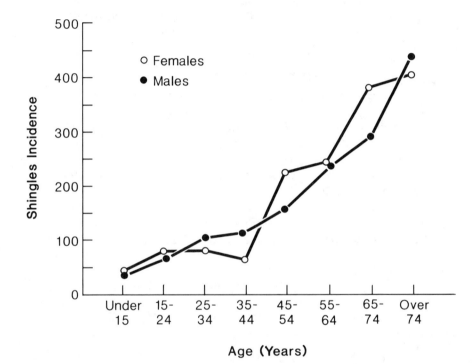

Incidence of shingles among a Rochester, Minnesota population. Shingles oc-
curs more frequently in older adults. The vertical scale is cases per 100,000 person-years.
Each year a patient is observed equals one person-year. M. W. Ragozzino et al., "Population-Based
Study of Herpes Zoster and Its Sequelae." *Medicine* 61 (1982):310-16. Reproduced with permission of the authors and
Williams and Wilkins Company.

who developed shingles on her face and nearly lost her job. Her employers equated herpes zoster with genital herpes and believed their children were threatened by a "social disease." Because of the unfortunate connotation of the medical term, our clinical virology staff refers to this disease as shingles or, occasionally, zoster, but never *herpes zoster*.

COURSE OF THE DISEASE

It felt like rain coming down on my head. — a Minneapolis man

Only my right side is affected — my right shoulder blade and my right rib cage. — a Kernville, Texas, man

If we have a hot summer I'll scratch my skin off. — a Taylors Falls, Minnesota, woman

The surface of the skin is so sensitive I can't even touch it. My doctor said I'll have to live with it. — a Toledo, Ohio, man

Where the Virus Hides

During our attack of childhood chickenpox, some virions escape the detection of our immune system by migrating to the dorsal root nerve ganglia along the spine. Dorsal root ganglia are collections of nerve cell bodies found along our back from the top of the spine, called cervical ganglia, to the bottom, named sacral. The varicella-zoster virus remains dormant for many years. Cancer patients receiving radiation treatments have provided evidence that many ganglia are seeded with virus during chickenpox. The site of their X ray therapy — no matter where — often erupts with shingles. Although many ganglia are infected during chickenpox, shingles usually results from reactivation of virions in one ganglion or several adjacent ganglia.

What Triggers an Attack

What causes varicella-zoster virus to erupt as shingles after remaining quiescent since our chickenpox attack in childhood? We are certain that cancer drugs, radiation treatments, and organ transplantation procedures trigger a shingles attack. In normal adults, emotional stress or physical trauma may reawaken the virus. Many of my patients say their shingles follows a life crisis such as divorce, death of a loved one, retirement, or a diagnosis of serious illness.

But still others can relate no additional stress or disruption in their life-style that might have triggered the dormant virus. In these cases, shingles may result from loss of immunologic memory. As people age, their immune recognition of a past infection fades. At a certain point the body can no longer keep the virus in check.

The earlier the age you experience chickenpox, the earlier you're likely to break out with shingles. This is especially true if infants develop chickenpox before they've lost their mother's transferred immunity. Maternal immunity does such a thorough job of clearing the infection that baby's white cells never "see" the virus. The baby's immune system cannot remember an invader it never encountered. Many of these children develop shingles before they enter elementary school!

Pain Followed by Rash

In most cases of acute shingles, a prodromal symptom—usually pain—precedes the rash. The exact cause of pain is unknown. We believe the pain is evidence of viral particles traveling away from a ganglion, where they have remained latent since the chickenpox attack, toward the skin. The tiny virions cause irritation and inflammation as they traverse the nerve. You may feel a very deep pain at first, since the virus is starting to move outward from deep within the back. After moving down nerve pathways, the virions leave nerve endings to infect skin cells, and the rash erupts.

Shingles patients commonly think their pain is caused by muscle irritation due to strenuous physical exercise. As a result, they may place a heating pad on the site of suspected injury. The ensuing rash is often attributed to a hot pad burn. Other patients think they are experiencing a heart attack or angina, and rush to a hospital emergency room or call the paramedics.

Rash develops two to three days after the onset of pain. The blisters form in croplike groupings, with as many as 40 to 50 tiny blisters in each patch of shingles. Shingles blistering is more severe than that of herpes simplex.

In normal individuals, the rash stays on one side of the body— either the left or the right. Why? Shingles virus usually reactivates from one ganglion. Ganglia along the spine are paired—one on the right and one on the left. For instance, ganglia on the left side of the spine have roots that extend from the center of the back around the left side of the body to the midline of our chest or abdomen. Nerve endings from left-sided ganglia don't cross over very far to the right. A typical patient whose virus reactivated from a left-sided ganglion near the top of the spine breaks out on the left upper back, under the left armpit, and across the left breast to the center of the rib cage.

Doctors say that the shingles rash has a "dermatome" distribution. A dermatome is a specific zone of sensation supplied by a nerve originating from one ganglion. Our dermatomes are indicated by the bands in the accompanying sketch. Shingles usually doesn't occupy the entire zone. The eruption is patchy, skipping large areas within the dermatome.

"Doctor, a neighbor told me that some people die if the rash wraps completely around their body. Is this so?" I have been asked this question at least a half-dozen times since the start of our shingles research. The answer is, of course, "No! In otherwise healthy people with normal immunity, the rash remains on one side of your body." Perhaps the myth of death by shingles originated in the experience of cancer patients who sometimes develop a disseminated rash, meaning that blisters cover much of the body on both the left and right sides. The patient eventually may die—because of cancer, not shingles.

The shingles rash evolves just like chickenpox: redness followed by papules (raised bumps). Within a day or two, papules fill with fluid and then are called vesicles (blisters). The vesicles turn from a clear to cloudy color as white blood cells move in to fight the virus. The cloudy material becomes thick pus, at which point the vesicles are termed pustules. The pustules solidify, crust, and the crusts or scabs eventually fall off. The healing process usually lasts two to three weeks.

Following an attack of shingles, patients may be left with slight discoloration of their skin. Skin texture may change too, becoming pitted at the site of the lesions. Scarring is unusual but can occur when the vesicles are very deep or become infected with bacteria. I advise patients to allow the rash to run its natural course. Resist scratching. Let the vesicles crust and dry in their own time.

The Wilmington, Delaware, woman who wrote our first excerpt described her shingles as "embarrassing." Some patients are concerned that shingles will be mistaken for herpes simplex, branding them as "loose" men or women. Other patients simply are upset by the unsightly rash, which they believe makes them ugly. One man told me, "I could hide my acne with flesh-colored ointment, but this shingles stuff is too much to disguise. I'll just have to stay at home awhile." My advice to patients is not to hide in the dark. Tell family and friends that shingles is a recurrence of chickenpox virus—not herpes. Then remember,

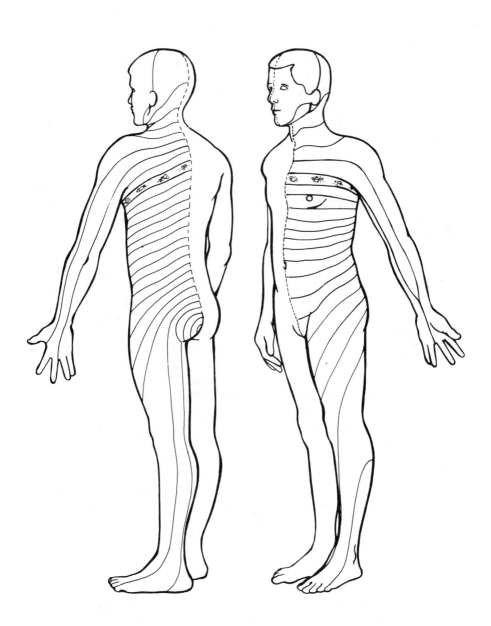

Dermatomes of the left side of the body, with shingles rash in one dermatome.

shingles (unlike acne) is temporary. Our face, the most visible place for shingles to attack, repairs itself much more rapidly than other parts of our body. Shingles on the face heals within 10 days in most patients.

Pain usually subsides as the rash heals. But some patients—about 10 percent—continue to have pain for months or years after their rash is gone. This condition, to be discussed later, is called postherpetic neuralgia.

Recurrences

Shingles rarely recurs. Of the 86 patients with normal immunity enrolled in three separate shingles studies at the University of Minnesota between 1980 and 1983, only two had recurrences. Recurrences may involve a different dermatome than the first outbreak.

Shingles in Immunosuppressed Patients

Patients who receive cancer treatment or antirejection medication following an organ transplant are more prone to a shingles attack because their immune systems are weakened. Until a decade ago, some medical textbooks said shingles was a sign of malignancy. That idea has been disproved. However, cancer patients have a greater probability of contracting shingles than others in their age-matched population. Patients with cancers involving the lymph glands, such as Hodgkin's disease, are especially vulnerable to shingles because they have only partial immunity to the virus. Their circulating T-lymphocytes don't recognize varicella-zoster virus. This defect is brought on by the tumor, not chemotherapy.

Most cancer patients handle shingles quite well. But a few—less than 1 percent—go on to develop involvement of lungs, liver, or central nervous system. Then, and only then, is the disease life threatening. The good news is that three drugs have been found to prevent shingles complications in immunosuppressed patients—vidarabine, interferon, and acyclovir. All three appear equally effective.

CONTAGIOUSNESS

Doctor, I just broke out in shingles. Can I attend my granddaughter's birthday party? —a St. Louis Park, Minnesota, woman

My receptionist has shingles involving the face. Her lesions crusted yesterday. We do see some pediatric patients. If she comes back to work, is there any risk of chickenpox? — a White Bear Lake, Minnesota, physician

I'm in my last trimester of pregnancy, and I just broke out in shingles on my side and chest. Will my baby catch chickenpox or shingles from me? — a University of Minnesota employee

Because shingles and chickenpox are caused by the same virus, exposure to shingles may cause chickenpox in someone (usually a child) who never had chickenpox before. If the shingles rash is covered by clothing—which is always the case unless the rash is on the face or hands—there is no risk of contagion. Once shingles has crusted, the patient cannot give a susceptible child chickenpox. Shingles patients are much less contagious than chickenpox sufferers because virus is present only in the shingles rash, not in the nose and mouth.

Shingles during pregnancy is not a problem for the baby. Maternal immunity limits shingles to the mother's affected nerves and skin. Virus will not cross the placenta to infect the infant before birth. The baby is in no danger after birth either. The newborn has sufficient maternal antibodies to destroy any virus acquired from contact with the mother's rash.

You will not catch shingles from a shingles patient. However, we have learned of several adults who developed shingles after exposure to chickenpox. The chickenpox exposure and subsequent shingles outbreak may have been coincidental. But there also may be a biological explanation. When our immune defense is invoked to fight the new varicella-zoster virions that are inhaled during an exposure to chickenpox, there may not be enough specific antibodies or knowledgeable lymphocytes left to keep the old virus, hiding in our nerve ganglia, in check. As the body is fending off the virus from the chickenpox contact, shingles erupts elsewhere.

CARE AND TREATMENT

I have a patient who has had pain for two weeks. Yesterday he broke out in shingles on the trunk. Would he be a good candidate for your study? — a St. Cloud, Minnesota, M.D.

I've been putting calamine lotion on my shingles. Is that a good idea? Will it help? — a Park Rapids, Minnesota, man

Home remedies for shingles abound because no specific treatment was available until very recently. Some simple things shingles sufferers can do for themselves are listed at the end of this section. And, at long last, a specific treatment—an antiviral drug against shingles—has arrived.

Development of New Drug against Shingles

In April 1981, we began experiments at the University of Minnesota to treat shingles with acyclovir. One of the major hurdles in developing a new treatment for any disease is finding patients. First, they must meet certain requirements regarding the severity of their illness. Second, they must be willing to accept either a placebo or a new therapy that might have harmful side effects.

There's a humorous proverb in medicine that goes, "It's hard to make a well patient better!" Applying this adage to clinical studies: a drug cannot be proved effective if patients are getting better before they take the test medicine. Many shingles patients are on the mend by the third or fourth day of rash. To give the new drug, acyclovir, a chance to work against shingles, we decided that therapy must begin within three days.

But how do you find patients whose disease is only three days old? Many individuals won't consult a doctor because of a peculiar rash until they've had it for a week or more. By that time, a physician's referral is too late. Therefore, we felt compelled to make public appeals via the news media to recruit patients.

In retrospect, I'm sure the Minneapolis-St. Paul press would have paid scant attention to shingles were it not caused by a member of the herpesvirus family. Thank heaven for relatives: reports that acyclovir was successful against herpes simplex directed newspapers, radio, and television to our doorstep. "We're testing acyclovir against another herpesvirus disease," we told them, "a disease more painful than cold sores or genital herpes."

As press coverage increased, so did our patient numbers. When the press lost interest, our recruitment efforts waned. Finally, we mailed letters to 4,500 Minnesota physicians. Our colleagues began searching for early cases of shingles, and the response was astounding! A sufficient number of patients were referred to us to complete our trial. When the results were analyzed, we learned that for the first time, a drug killed varicella-zoster virus in normal adults, resulting in pain relief for patients in the early stages of their shingles. Here is a summary of the findings that my colleague Dr. Bonnie Bean, our research nurse Carol

Braun, and I published in the July 17, 1982, issue of an international medical journal, *Lancet*:

• Pain in patients who received intravenous acyclovir subsided significantly faster than pain in the placebo group during the five-day study. Median time for reduction in pain was two days for acyclovir recipients and five days for those receiving placebo.

• Blister healing in the acyclovir group occurred an average of two days after treatment was started, compared with five days in placebo recipients.

• The antiviral drug prevented the formation of new lesions.

• A smaller percentage of acyclovir patients had postherpetic neuralgia compared with their placebo counterparts, but the difference was not statistically significant.

Specific antiviral therapy is now available for shingles in the form of acyclovir injections. But many shingles patients are not sick enough to require frequent intravenous medication. Since acyclovir tablets have not yet been shown effective against shingles, we're still awaiting specific practical treatment. In the meantime, patients can manage shingles by themselves.

Tips on Managing Acute Shingles

• Practice good personal hygiene. Washing the affected area daily with soap and water protects damaged skin from bacterial infection.

• Using a face cloth dipped in lukewarm saltwater (one teaspoon of salt per quart) as a compress, gently cover the blisters for periods of five to 10 minutes two to three times a day. Except for applying compresses, leave the rash alone. Ointments and creams are of no benefit.

• Try aspirin or acetaminophen for pain and itching. If necessary, your doctor may prescribe something stronger.

• Relax. Do as little as possible for a few days. Reducing work and any stress-related activities may shorten your illness.

Do Steriods Help?

The doctors have treated me with steroids without success. I have been to four doctors. None could help. I have had seven nerve blocks. Nothing helps. —a South Bend, Indiana, man

Steroids have been painted on the shingles rash, injected into the rash, and given by mouth. Steroid medications resemble natural hormones secreted by our adrenal glands. The major effect of steroids is to reduce inflammation—but in so doing they are immunosuppressive. We want our immune defense to be at its strongest against varicella-zoster virus. Weakening the immune system by using steroids is not sensible. Furthermore, steroids have no effect on skin healing or pain during the first few weeks of shingles.

Because two earlier studies suggest that steroids might reduce the incidence and duration of postherpetic neuralgia, Dr. Richard Whitley of the University of Alabama is investigating the role of steroids in shingles management. Until his results are available, I do not recommend routine use of steroids for shingles.

POSTHERPETIC NEURALGIA

Regardless of any kind of treatment, my husband's face and head are very sore and hurt all of the time. He can't stand wind on his face and eye. It hurts him to put his hat on. —a Centertown, Missouri, woman

I have had every treatment and procedure known today, with no permanent relief. You name it and I've had it, including intravenous injections of DMSO. The results were not worth it. I am now taking methadone every four hours for relief. The pain is getting progressively worse and more constant, and it has now come to where I can hardly stay on my feet for any length of time. —a Laguna Hills, California, woman

I have had 30 treatments of acupuncture, and it has not helped at all. There has been talk of clipping the nerves in the area. I have seen three neurosurgeons and have been to a major teaching hospital, and have had no results. —a New York City woman

An acute disease lasts only a short time, usually less than a month. The initial episode of shingles is referred to as an acute attack. For most patients, shingles is over in two to three weeks. But some continue to suffer from the painful aftereffects of the disease, called postherpetic neuralgia. These individuals are considered chronic sufferers. *Chronic* is defined as an illness of long duration, always longer than a month.

Ten percent of all zoster patients experience postherpetic neuralgia—a persistent pain that lasts months or years after the shingles attack. Neuralgia rarely occurs in patients under the age of 50. But the incidence increases drastically as age at onset of shingles increases. In the Rochester, Minnesota, study cited earlier, Dr. M. W. Ragozzino reported that the average age of patients with postherpetic neuralgia was 67, compared with 46 for patients whose pain resolved during acute shingles.

My correspondence came primarily from patients and relatives struggling with neuralgia. Their emotion-filled letters tell the story better than any medical textbook. They certainly would convince my young medical friend that shingles is no joke. Sometimes you can almost feel the pain in the styling of the words. Several writers obviously made a great physical effort just to pen a brief letter. The pain is most often described as a "knife turning inside," "a burning like I had picked up a hot plate, but it won't stop." Because the pain won't cease, neuralgia victims have great difficulty sleeping and performing daily tasks. Their lives become obsessed with coping—just existing—with pain.

Two theories have been advanced to explain the cause of postherpetic neuralgia. The first school of thought contends that sensory nerves are permanently damaged as virions travel from the ganglia to the skin during the acute shingles attack. The second hypothesis suggests that a low level of viral replication continues long after the acute shingles attack subsides. This is akin to the trickle theory of herpes simplex recurrence. Quite possibly, varicella-zoster virions are continually raining down the nerve pathways, causing constant inflammation and pain.

If the virus remains active, we should be able to find viral remnants in nerve tissues of patients with postherpetic neuralgia. We are investigating this hypothesis at the University of Minnesota. A neurosurgeon removes a small segment of intercostal nerve that courses between the ribs in the area of the patient's neuralgia. This biopsied tissue is processed in the laboratory, where a scientist looks for miniscule pieces of varicella-zoster virus.

What might this study mean for patients? If the theory of persistent viral activity is correct, antiviral drugs may hasten resolution of pain by killing the live virus. On the other hand, if irreparable nerve damage has occurred and virus is not present, antiviral therapy will be of no help.

Postherpetic neuralgia gradually dissipates in many patients. We can only hypothesize why. Nerves from their cell bodies near the spine to endings in the skin are damaged during an acute shingles attack. Pain may be the result of nerve cell damage. The nerves have a limited ability to repair themselves, however. Once the nerve cell bodies and their extensions have healed, painful sensations may cease. Another possibility is that damage to nerve cells results from continuous multiplication of virus in the neurons or adjacent supporting cells. Eventually our immune system rids us of all new virions, and the painful damage resolves.

Research is proceeding on the premise that early treatment of acute shingles may reduce the risk of chronic neuralgia. Logic tells us that if we can eradicate the virions before large numbers climb inside nerve cells, they will wreak less havoc on nerve tissue.

MANAGEMENT OF POSTHERPETIC NEURALGIA

I need help soon because my next step is suicide. I am 69 years old and have had three different doctors, and they all said I will have to live with this herpes zoster for the next two years. I am going mad with the pain and will not last that long. — a St. Petersburg, Florida, man

I saw a dermatologist who said he treats postherpetic neuralgia. So he gave me an injection in the area under my arm—that was in June of this year—no relief. He gave me other medications . . . and no results. So he told me to come back in November when he would give me something stronger. But my medical doctor thinks he put me off—because he didn't have anything. — a Toledo, Ohio, woman

I had an implant of an electronic device attached to my spine running to an implanted coil to which I have attached a transmitter that is supposed to help block out my pain. Because of the soreness of the various incisions, I am not fully able to ascertain if it will entirely block my pain, but from what I have found out thus far, I believe that it will block the sharpness from the pains that I am experiencing. —a Linton, Indiana, man

Can you imagine pain so terrible that you want to die? The common thread among all shingles patients, especially those with postherpetic neuralgia, is severe, unrelenting pain. Unless you are a victim, it may be hard to understand their plight. A Minneapolis neurologist, ranking pain on a scale of one to 10, rates migraine headache a four, passing kidney stones a nine, and shingles a six and a half or seven. Shingles pain is usually constant.

Don Boxmeyer, a writer for the *St. Paul Dispatch* newspaper, related his shingles experience in an August 27, 1983, column entitled "Shingles: Baffling Ailment Traps Upper Torso in Waves of Pain." He wrote, in part:

Among the worst experiences when the pain was at its height was the simple act of putting a shirt on; it was something like rubbing sand-paper against a sunburn. I also discovered that the breeze from an electric fan against skin was like having a 15-pound cat crawl up my back.

The medical debate about treatment of pain has raged for many years. How often and how potent a pain-killing drug do we give the patient? What is worse: enduring the pain or risking drug addiction? Some doctors prefer to keep their patients off pain medication at all costs. I believe analgesics including narcotics are appropriate therapy for acute shingles pain. Chronic sufferers must be managed differently, perhaps with only occasional use of analgesics; otherwise the pain medications lose their desired effect. We call this developing a tolerance for the medications.

There is no proven treatment for postherpetic neuralgia. As you can see from the many excerpts in this chapter, victims have tried everything. Of course, those who wrote us did not represent a true cross section of shingles sufferers because we heard from the patients whose therapy did not work. Perhaps acupuncture or another technique helped others.

How can you deal with the pain of postherpetic neuralgia? This difficult question usually is posed by an elderly individual, who probably has other medical problems. Such patients are in a state of confusion, fear, and even anger at the medical profession for not offering an answer.

The following suggestions come from patients who are successfully *managing* their postherpetic neuralgia:

• Try to accept your pain. That may sound trite, condescending, and downright impossible. But patients who seem to be tolerating postherpetic neuralgia best are those who realize that pain is a reality of life. Says one patient: "I've had the pain for two years; I can't expect it will go away in two weeks."

• Develop relationships with people who share your predicament. On one occasion, two of my neuralgia patients met in our clinic and struck up an immediate friendship when they realized that they both had the same terrible pain. I overheard one man say, "No one else understands."

• Consult a physician who has experience with shingles and pain therapy.

• Do relaxation exercises. If your pain comes in waves and you have an idea when it is about to begin, learn breathing techniques. Concentration on breathing may alleviate the intensity of the attack.

- Apply ice packs. They offer temporary relief for some.
- Consult a physical therapist. Our program makes frequent referrals to physical therapists who will advise you on exercise, breathing, relaxation techniques.
- Hypnosis, acupuncture, and nerve stimulation do not help everyone, but no two people are identical. They may help you.

How Others May Help You: Two Stories
Lonely and isolated people seem to have the most difficulty coping. In their waning years of life, elderly men and women may have little else on which to concentrate except their pain. Here are two patients whose attitudes toward pain are very different because of their environment.

One of our suicide threats came from a St. Paul woman named Lucille, a 62-year-old widow who lives alone, has no children and few friends. Postherpetic neuralgia so incapacitated her that she gave up her business as an antique dealer. Except for a two-hour shopping trip every morning, she spends the rest of the day closeted in her house, wearing only a light, loose-fitting cotton gown to reduce friction on her body.

In contrast, Howard lives in a house full of grandchildren, where activity is constant. Some of the children even accompany him to our clinic. Howard once told me, "The neuralgia hurts, of course, but my family keeps my mind on other things."

We can't compare the intensity of Lucille's pain with Howard's. Objective methods to measure pain are not available. But psychologically, there's no question that Howard has a better outlook on life because he can share his predicament with others.

COMPLICATIONS

My sister-in-law has had shingles and complications since March 1981. She is disfigured and can't read because one eye is forever clouded. —a Tucson, Arizona, woman

I was treated for an ulcer in the left eye. Needless to say, I lost much of my sight. The left eye is cloudy and feels like there's a film over it. I still have the quivering or tingling on the left side of my face. —a Chippewa Falls, Wisconsin, man

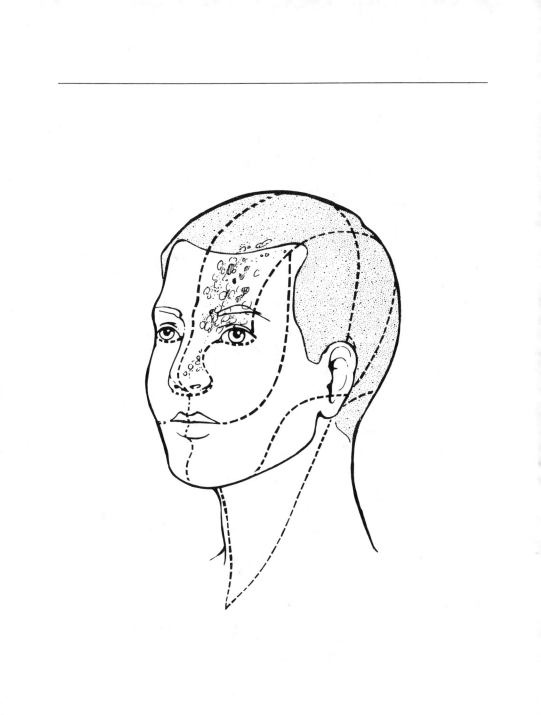

Shingles invading a facial dermatome. When present in this dermatome, the eye is often affected.

The shingles has affected my right hand and right arm. I have definite tremors. —a East Hartford, Connecticut, woman

Shingles has several complications besides postherpetic neuralgia. About 5 percent of all patients suffer either generalized skin rash or central nervous system involvement including encephalitis.

The most common of the serious complications of acute shingles is scarring of the eye. About 20 percent of shingles patients have zoster on the face. In these cases, virions have migrated to the skin via the fifth cranial nerve, called the trigeminal nerve, which has three branches— one of them being the ophthalmic branch. If virions invade the ophthalmic branch, they can reach the eye. The eye becomes infected in about 50 percent of all cases of facial shingles. The cornea is most frequently affected and can be scarred. I recommend that any patient who has shingles on the face see an ophthalmologist.

Shingles sometimes interferes with muscle function, as reported by the Connecticut woman. Virions normally move along the sensory nerve pathways, but occasionally go off course, afflicting motor nerves to cause tremors or paralysis.

CONCLUSION: EARLY TREATMENT—BEST RESULTS

Unless I can get results, I don't feel like I can waste my money for treatments that don't help. —a Dayton, Ohio, woman

I certainly agree with this Ohio woman that nostrums aren't worth the money and trouble. But now, a specific treatment for new cases of shingles has been discovered. The best outcome seems to follow early treatment. Consult a physician at once if a painful rash erupts on one side of your body. Clinical research has proved that antiviral drugs shorten the acute pain. I firmly believe that when more results are in, early treatment also will be shown to prevent postherpetic neuralgia.

Mono Virus and the Cancer Connection

Can you imagine a more frightening thought than "catching" cancer from a kiss? In fact, until 1920, the ailment now known as the "kissing disease" or infectious mononucleosis was believed to be acute leukemia. Because the early stages of leukemia may mimic mononucleosis, doctors had great difficulty differentiating between the two. A patient's return to good health was often attributed to a spontaneous remission of leukemia.

The scientists who first identified the mono virus now named after them—M. Anthony Epstein and Yvonne Barr—were actually involved in cancer research when they made their discovery in 1964. Today, two decades after Epstein-Barr virus (EBV) became the "official" name for the mono bug, researchers are finding new evidence that this virus not only causes mono but is indeed linked to cancer.

TRACING A DISEASE—HISTORICAL MEDICINE

Patient H. C., Medical No. 31625. White woman, unmarried. Age: 23 years. Medical Student. Admitted to the hospital October 24, 1913. Discharged November 18, 1913. Acute febrile disease without local manifestations except marked lymphocytosis and enlargement of lymph nodes and spleen. Recovery.

In 1920, Drs. Thomas Sprunt and Frank Evans of Johns Hopkins University and Hospital analyzed the cases of six young patients, including H. C., in what became the first clinical description of a new disease called infectious mononucleosis. Of course, doctors had seen patients with similar symptoms (high fever, swollen glands, malaise) before 1920. Sprunt and Evans wrote, "Although these reports have been in the literature for some time, such cases are not very generally recognized [as infectious mononucleosis] and each new one is apt to give rise to grave apprehension of the onset of a leukemia state."

Historical accounts of infectious mononucleosis date to the late

1880s when German and Russian scientists, working independently, described patients with high fever, enlarged lymph glands, malaise, and abdominal pain. The Germans called the illness Drusenfieber for glandular swelling, but they had no test to differentiate Drusenfieber, which seemed to appear frequently in certain families, from cancer. As the Drusenfieber concept fell into disrepute, the idea of spontaneous remission of cancer gained popularity.

Sprunt and Evans were the first to provide doctors with a method of distinguishing between cancer and infectious mononucleosis. In studying blood smears of their patients, they found very large leukocytes (white cells) with a single nucleus (called mononuclear cells, hence the name mononucleosis) that differed from leukemia cells. There was an excess of these unusual lymphocytes in the bloodstream. The medical term for such an increase is lymphocytosis. A full page color plate illustrating the distinctive features of mononucleosis leukocytes accompanied Sprunt and Evans' report in the *Johns Hopkins Hospital Bulletin* to help pathologists make the correct diagnosis. At that time, color plates were used sparsely, and only for significant medical findings. This was, unquestionably, an important medical achievement.

Although the Johns Hopkins scientists provided a "clear cut clinical picture" of infectious mononucleosis, they were unable to identify a cause. A virus found in a malignant tumor more than 40 years later was shown subsequently and serendipitously to be the culprit.

At Middlesex Hospital in London in the early 1960s, Epstein, a pathologist, and Barr, his chief assistant, were studying biopsy specimens from patients with an unusual tumor of lymphocytes called Burkitt's lymphoma. Using the electron microscope, they observed tiny herpesvirus particles inside the cancer cells. Their findings, presented in 1964, marked the discovery of Epstein-Barr virus, the newest member of the human herpesvirus family.

A serendipitous event occurred four years later when a technologist working in the laboratory of Drs. Werner and Gertrude Henle at Children's Hospital of Philadelphia was stricken with infectious mononucleosis. Because the Henles had been studying Burkitt's lymphoma, looking for evidence of the causative virus in Americans, some of the tech's blood had been tested and stored. When they examined this previously collected sample and others taken during the mono illness, they found EBV in the leukocytes and a diagnostic rise in EBV antibodies. Such was the conclusive identification of EBV as the "mono virus."

HOW THE DISEASE SPREADS

Armed for the first time with a specific test for mononucleosis, scientists now could investigate the natural history of mono in various population groups firsthand. Both American and British investigators launched epidemiological studies.

The West Point Study

In July 1969, one year after it was confirmed that EBV causes mononucleosis, the entire entering class of 1,401 cadets at the U.S. Military Academy at West Point, New York, became research subjects in one of the most thorough epidemiological investigations of infectious mononucleosis ever undertaken. The cadets constituted a nearly ideal study group because they represented a cross section of young adults from across the United States, were in the most mono-prone period of their lives, and could be followed closely for a specific period.

The study, conducted by researchers at Yale University School of Medicine and the New York State Health Department, provided detailed information on mono's prevalence (the number of cadets with EBV antibody at any one time), incidence (number of new infections in a given period), symptoms, and contagiousness.

Upon arrival at the Academy, the cadets completed medical history forms that included questions designed to detect a previous bout of mononucleosis. Their blood was checked for EBV antibody. During the next four years, all the cadets were observed for infectious mononucleosis or any illness with similar symptoms. Blood samples were taken annually and results correlated with hospital records.

On entry into the study, 63.5 percent of the cadets possessed EBV antibody whereas 36.5 percent showed no sign of previous EBV infection. At the end of the four-year study, researchers offered the following observations:

• About half of the cadets who lacked EBV antibody when they arrived at West Point and who were followed for at least a year (201 of 437) were infected with the virus during their four-year college experience.

• Only 26.4 percent of the 201 newly infected cadets had a recognized episode of infectious mononucleosis.

• EBV infections were *not* more common in exposed, susceptible (no EBV antibody) roommates than in the susceptible cadet population whose roommates did not contract mono.

• Except for two cadets already ill at the time of their initial blood

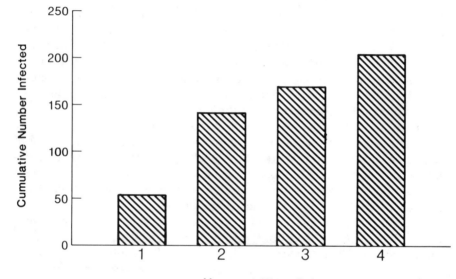

Incidence of infectious mononucleosis among 437 susceptible West Point cadets. Source: T. J. Hallee et al. "Infectious Mononucleosis at the United States Military Academy: A Prospective Study of a Single Class over Four Years." *Yale Journal of Biology and Medicine* 3 (1974):182–95.

check, infectious mononucleosis was not observed in any of the 890 cadets possessing EBV antibody on entry. In other words, there were no symptomatic recurrences of infectious mono. (More on this later.)

The West Point study documented, for the first time, the rate of infection during the college-age years. Mononucleosis spreads rapidly among young adults. On the average, 20 percent of the susceptible cadets experienced a virus attack every year.

The cadets' study shed light on *how* EBV is caught. If EBV were airborne like flu, roommates would catch mono. Because the susceptible roommates didn't, we had evidence that acquisition of EBV required more than simply being together in the same room. The study indirectly supported the common concept that mono is the kissing disease after all.

The report also provided insight into the relative severity of infectious mononucleosis. More than half of the infected cadets showed no signs of illness or experienced mild nondescript symptoms. In other words, many cases of infectious mononucleosis resembled the common cold. These cadets were ill, but not sick enough to seek medical help. If they had, their doctor could have ordered a lab test to diagnose the mono infection.

An English Study Confirms U.S. Findings

Meanwhile, researchers in Great Britain reported strikingly similar findings from their study of 1,457 students who entered five English colleges and universities in October 1969. Blood tests upon matriculation revealed that 55 percent of freshmen from the British Isles already possessed EBV antibody. A retest seven months later found that an additional 12 percent had acquired the antibody. Of these newly infected students, about one-third showed no sign of illness; one-fifth had mild respiratory ailments; and nearly half had experienced typical infectious mononucleosis.

The scientists concluded in the *British Medical Journal*, December 11, 1971:

> *The results of this study leave no doubt . . . that many British students already have EB virus antibody by the time they enter university (55%). An even greater rate (84%) was observed in students from tropical countries. Probably this antibody usually develops without overt infectious mononucleosis since it is rarely diagnosed in children.*

Evidently EB virus antibody is acquired by many students early in college life; indeed the findings during seven months would give an annual incidence of about 20 percent. If this rate were to continue, about three-quarters of all students would have antibody to the virus by the time they leave university. These findings, provided they are generally applicable, would explain the low incidence of infectious mononucleosis among older persons in Britain.

WHAT THE PATIENTS SAY—TWO CASE REPORTS

The incidence of mononucleosis is highest in the 15-to-25-year age group. Two young adults who came down with full blown mono tell their stories this way:

Kim: "I Looked Like Twiggy"

I was 17 years old, a high school senior, and captain of my cheerleading squad. On the morning after a particularly exciting football game, I awoke with a scratchy throat. I assumed it was due to hoarseness because I had done lots of cheering. But by Saturday night I felt weak, and Mom noted a slight fever. So I was sent to bed and slept until midday Sunday. When Mom found my temperature had reached 102 degrees, she phoned the doctor, who prescribed aspirin and scheduled a clinic appointment for the next morning. By the time of the visit, my sore throat was almost unbearable. I was still weak and had a stomachache. After a short examination, the doctor said he believed that I was suffering from a classic case of infectious mononucleosis. He said the stomachache could be due to enlargement of my spleen, packed with white cells rallying to fight infection. The doctor prescribed bed rest, aspirin for my headache, and lozenges for my sore throat. He said he couldn't be sure, but warned me that I would probably miss several weeks of school. He also asked to be kept advised of any improvement or worsening in my condition.

I was really scared by my illness. I slept so much that I set my clock every night, even though I didn't have to, because I was afraid that I wouldn't wake up. I returned to school four weeks later, just in time for the last football game of the season. I felt a little tired before the game, but it was my last chance to cheerlead. The next day I was back in bed, exhausted, aching all over. I missed about 10 more days of school, and when I went back the second time I forced myself to slow down to make sure I didn't get sick again. I lost about 15 pounds, dropping from 125 to 110. Friends said I looked like Twiggy when I returned to school. I'd planned to lose some weight, but this was too much!

Comment: Kim is representative of the 25 to 50 percent of patients who develop recognizable mononucleosis following EBV infection: rapid onset of symptoms followed by several weeks of rest before recovery. Like many others, Kim attempted to return to a normal schedule of activity—studies, exercise, and other tasks—before she was totally well. As a result, she suffered a relapse. Doctors cannot provide a specific timetable for recovery.

Charlie's Brush with "Leukemia"

I was 24 years old when I developed infectious mononucleosis, but I thought I was dying of leukemia because of a bizarre-looking blood smear which I misdiagnosed. I was in my second year of medical school, struggling through several strenuous courses that required more than 20 hours of laboratory work each week. I awoke one morning feeling run down. I had no fever, no chills, no sore throat. The next day, I felt even worse—like I had a hangover—although I hadn't been drinking. Everything I did was an effort, but somehow I managed to make it to class.

Coincidentally, my hematology class was studying the morphology (appearance) of circulating blood cells. One of our laboratory exercises was to compare blood samples with our classmates. You would finger-stick your lab partner with a lancet, smear a thin film of blood on a glass slide, stain it, and examine the cells under a microscope. My lab mate's blood was textbook normal, but mine looked horrible! I was afraid to say anything to my instructor.

I hurried back to my dorm and reread the chapter on leukemia in my pathology text. The next day, convinced I had leukemia, I timidly approached the hematology professor in charge of the class and showed him my blood sample. What a relief when he exclaimed, "Charlie, you do have abnormal cells, but they aren't leukemic. Those are Downey cells, characteristic of infectious mononucleosis."

I became steadily sicker during the next two to three weeks. I was weak, with a terrible headache and funny burning sensations in my arms and legs. I later learned that the virus can actually enter the central nervous system. I also became depressed because the mono was jeopardizing my medical studies. Somehow, I managed to struggle through the semester. I was in bed every night by nine o'clock and got out of the sack just in time to grab a bite of breakfast before class. My appetite was off for about two months. I didn't feel like my normal, active self for at least six months. It was a tiring experience—both physically and emotionally.

Comment: Some mono blood smears look malignant, even to the experienced pathologist. About 1 percent of mono patients have neurological symptoms. Charlie's were called paresthesias, which are unreal perceptions such as a burning sensation when nothing is there to cause heat.

HOW THE DISEASE IS CAUGHT

Only 6 percent of patients can recall prior contact with a mono sufferer. So how do the majority of us catch the virus?

EBV lingers in the throat long after a mono attack. Transmission most frequently occurs during intimate contact between the asymptomatic EBV carriers and susceptible individuals. The virus can be passed in saliva—thus the term kissing disease—or in blood or blood products. Because mono is sometimes blood-borne, the American Association of Blood Banks recommends that member facilities not accept blood from donors who report a mono infection during the previous six months. There is no evidence that EBV is transmitted through genital contact.

The typical incubation period lasts 30 to 60 days. EBV can survive in the throat up to 18 months after clinical recovery from mono. The virus remains very much alive during this period, capable of contaminating anyone who comes into contact with it. Interestingly, 10 to 20 percent of healthy adults shed virus from the throat. This means that asymptomatic recurrences are common. Like other members of the herpesvirus family, EBV does not survive very long on inanimate surfaces.

College students and military servicemen have the greatest incidence of infectious mononucleosis, probably the result of numerous heterosexual experiences during their late teens and early twenties. Lower socioeconomic groups have a higher prevalence of EBV antibody, indicating exposure to the virus (perhaps due to crowded living conditions) during early childhood when the clinical expression of mono is quite mild. This is similar to what happens with herpes simplex type 1, as we've seen in chapter 4.

COURSE AND COMPLICATIONS

Typical mononucleosis has a triad of symptoms: sore throat, fever, and enlarged lymph glands in the neck. Patients also report chills, malaise, nausea, abdominal discomfort, vomiting, and loss of appetite. A few victims become jaundiced, indicating that virus has invaded their liver and compromised liver function.

The onset of mono is usually abrupt, although many patients identify prodromal symptoms such as chills, sweats, or fever. Smokers commonly lose their taste for cigarettes.

If you or someone in your family has these symptoms, I recommend seeing your doctor who can confirm or rule out mono. Physicians base the diagnosis on physical findings, examination of a blood smear for mononucleosis cells, and other laboratory studies including a heterophile test, mono spot test, and measurement of antibodies specifically directed against EBV.

Mono usually lasts two to six weeks. Sore throat is noticeable for seven to 10 days but is most painful for the first three to five days. Fever persists for 10 to 14 days, then gradually abates. Malaise and weakness may linger for months. Uncommon complications include rupture of the spleen, respiratory difficulty due to swollen tonsils and adenoids, anemia, and encephalitis.

Generally speaking, the older the individual at the onset of EBV infection, the more severe the illness. In children, the primary infection usually goes undetected. Patients who have the greatest difficulty coping are adolescents and young adults. It is unusual for older adults to develop mono, probably because of their monogamous life style and immunity developed over time.

Mono during Pregnancy

EBV infections occur during pregnancy, but the developing fetus rarely is injured. A few babies suffer birth defects associated with maternal mono during gestation. These include abnormalities of the central nervous system, congenital heart disease, and bone deformities. As a sensible precaution, I advise pregnant women not to kiss anyone who has had infectious mononucleosis within the past three months.

Relapses

Relapses are frequent because many patients attempt to return to a normal level of activity before they are totally well. *Relapse* means worsening of the present illness. In contrast, *recurrence* is a renewal of symptoms after the initial illness has completely healed. Recurrences of mono are uncommon; the West Point study did not document a single recurrence among the military cadets during their four years at the Academy.

The Immortalization of Mono Virus

EBV attacks B-lymphocytes, fitting snugly on their outer surface like the right piece of a jigsaw puzzle. After attachment, EBV quickly penetrates the cell membrane and eventually enters the nucleus. The B-cells then become "immortalized" because once infected, they survive forever, keeping EBV alive within them. As a result, EBV, like other members of the herpesvirus family, never totally leaves our body.

EBV frequently reactivates from the latent state in B-lymphocytes, but the episodes go unrecognized. Are reactivations important, then? Yes. Transmission of EBV is facilitated when the virus reactivates in the throat of an unknowing carrier who then kisses an unsuspecting victim. Reactivation of EBV can be a serious consequence for organ transplant patients who had mono as young adults. These patients can experience a recurrence of mono after transplantation or the virus can lead to something more malignant (see the section on the virus-cancer link later in this chapter).

CARE AND TREATMENT

A number of measures are helpful during the acute illness:

• For severe sore throats: gargle with warm salt water to reduce swelling; drink a liberal amount of liquid; eat light foods like jello, popsicles, ice cream, soups, and broth; use throat lozenges for short-term relief; take aspirin or acetaminophen, or a stronger pain medication if prescribed.

• Avoid alcoholic beverages during the acute phase of the disease because mono always attacks the liver to some degree. Alcohol is a liver toxin, and the combination of infection and toxin may damage that vital organ.

• Steroids may lessen the intensity and duration of symptoms, but a physician should exercise good judgment in prescribing them because of their possible side effects. Remember that steroids suppress immunity—and a strong immune defense is vital for ridding us of mono.

• There is no need for isolation precautions because the virus is spread only by intimate contact.

• Resume a normal routine *slowly*. If you increase your activities too rapidly, as Kim did, you may wind up back in bed.

• When you feel fit enough, it's okay to date. But out of consideration for your companion, avoid mouth-to-mouth contact, especially French kissing, for at least two months.

Drugs against the mono virus are now being developed and tested in patients. Results are inconclusive so far.

THE VIRUS-CANCER LINK

In 1978, while working on the transplant service at University of Minnesota Hospitals, second-year surgical resident Dr. Douglas Hanto was assigned the task of compiling statistics on kidney transplant patients who developed cancer. His purpose: to determine risk factors for acquiring cancer after transplantation. The project may have seemed mundane for an aspiring surgeon, but there was no question of the importance of the job.

The specter of cancer has haunted transplant surgeons and immunologists since a correlation was first noted between cancer and kidney transplantation in 1969. After receiving a new kidney, patients are one hundred times more likely to develop cancer than others of the same age in the population at large. Overall, about 6 percent of posttransplant patients get cancer.

One of Hanto's patients was a 60-year-old man who had received a cadaver kidney transplant in 1970. He was rehospitalized in April 1978 after an eight-week bout with a very sore throat. The patient's condition was much more serious than a throat infection. A biopsy revealed a tumor on the base of his tongue; the lesion was classified as a malignant lymphoma.

Lymphoma, a cancer of the lymphatic system, accounts for 20 percent of all posttransplant malignancies. This form of cancer typically begins in a lymph gland and quickly spreads to the body's vital organs. It is almost always fatal in transplant patients.

"There were some unusual things about this patient, however," Hanto said. "First, the tumor began in his mouth, which is atypical in transplant patients. He also had some characteristics that resembled mononucleosis." Acting on a hunch, Hanto ordered antibody tests on his patient for the mono virus. Tests confirmed an acute EBV infection!

Investigators had hypothesized for years that cancer after transplantation was virus-induced; some even suspected EBV to be the culprit. But none had been able to provide supporting evidence. This was due to several reasons: transplant patients were scarce; clinical features of the tumors were not well defined; the pathology (tissue changes due to disease) was confusing; and the cancers were called by five or six different names.

The surgical residency program at Minnesota gave Hanto a unique opportunity to probe deeper into the transplant-cancer mystery. In addition to various rotations in the operating room, transplant residents are required to spend at least two years doing basic laboratory research. Because of the striking findings in the 60-year-old transplant patient, and his own curiosity, Hanto decided to focus on the transplant-cancer-EBV enigma during the research phase of his surgical fellowship.

Collaborating with researchers in pathology, immunology, and virology, Hanto and colleagues discovered that two patients had multiple copies of the EBV DNA in their tumors, strong evidence linking EBV with posttransplant cancer. Hanto's study, published in the March 1981 issue of the journal *Transplantation Proceedings*, concluded that "EBV is implicated as [a cancer] inducing agent in the immunosuppressed transplant patient."

Next, a most surprising twist in the EBV-cancer story was reported in the *New England Journal of Medicine* in April 1982. Hanto and fellow scientists described the case of a 12-year-old transplant patient whose recurrent tumors associated with acute EBV infection responded to antiviral therapy. I'll call this patient "Jerry."

Transplant Drama

Jerry received a kidney transplant from his mother in November 1977. Because of chronic rejection, the organ had to be removed 19 months later. Jerry then received a cadaver kidney in January 1980. About four months later, Jerry was readmitted because of soaking night sweats and a strange buildup of tissue around his ear. A biopsy of the tissue revealed a cancerous condition known as "polymorphic B-cell lymphoma." Surprisingly, further tests showed that more than 80 percent of the cells were infected with EBV.

Based on our previous experience with other transplant patients who had similar tumors, we knew that Jerry's chances were slim and that only extraordinary measures would save his life. We therefore embarked on a treatment plan that involved reducing the immunosuppressive drugs used to fight rejection because they limited the body's natural efforts to combat the cancer. We also started injections of an experimental antiviral drug, acyclovir, to fight the virus.

Jerry received intravenous acyclovir for seven days. He began to show signs of improvement after only three days. His fever dropped and he resumed normal activity. A repeat biopsy performed at the end of the seven-day course of acyclovir showed fewer cancer cells in the boy's body. But 48 hours after treatment concluded, Jerry's fever returned, he felt weak, and lost his appetite. The antiviral drug therapy was restarted and again led to dramatic resolution of the fever. He was discharged with no more signs of cancer.

About six months after transplantation, Jerry experienced acute rejection of the donor kidney, necessitating a significant increase in his immunosuppressive drugs. Four weeks later he was rehospitalized with fever, sore throat, swollen tonsils, and enlarged lymph glands in his neck. A biopsy of the tonsils and involved lymph glands was interpreted as B-cell lymphoma. And, again, 80 percent of the cells showed the presence of EBV. Acyclovir therapy was given for two weeks; the lymph gland swelling regressed but did not disappear. He continued to suffer from many of the same symptoms. Two months later he was given a final course of acyclovir without benefit. He died a short time later.

Comment: Although Jerry's story ended tragically, the case provided scientists with information that may save others from this unfortunate consequence of transplantation. During its early phase, Jerry's specific kind of cancer responded to an antiviral drug, suggesting, perhaps for the first time, that a herpesvirus infection was aiding and abetting a cancerous growth. Stopping that viral infection caused regression of the tumor on at least two occasions, but in the end the cancerous cells no longer needed EBV for sustenance. The antiviral drug bought some time for Jerry, but that was all. The war against the tumor was lost. If Jerry's embattled immune state had not been further weakened by antirejection therapy, perhaps the tumor's growth could have been held in check.

Ensuing studies on 19 kidney transplant patients demonstrated that EBV causes a spectrum of lymphoproliferative diseases ranging from infectious mononucleosis to malignant lymphomas. These Minnesota patients offered supporting evidence for the long-standing hypothesis of an EBV-cancer connection. Researchers Epstein and Barr, as you recall, were involved in cancer research when they first identified the virus in patients with Burkitt's lymphoma in 1964.

Burkitt's lymphoma involves facial bones, ovaries, and abdominal lymph tissue. Although rarely seen in the Western world, the cancer frequently strikes children in Africa. Nearly every African patient with Burkitt's lymphoma possesses high antibody titers to EBV. However, very few African children with EBV antibody suffer from Burkitt's lymphoma, implying that other factors, such as a genetic predisposition or an environmental carcinogen, must also be involved in the triggering of the cancer. The fact that Burkitt's lymphoma is rare in the United States whereas EBV infections are common gives credence to the multicause theory. To confound matters further, in most cases of Burkitt's in the United States there is no evidence of EBV in tumor cells.

Burkitt's was the first but not the only tumor to be associated with EBV. Nasopharyngeal carcinoma, a cancer of the nose, nasal passages, and pharynx, has also been tied to EBV. This cancer is prevalent among African and Oriental groups but rarely found in Europe and the United States.

Why is EBV the herpes family member most closely connected with human cancer? Normal circulating lymphocytes do not divide, and their life is spent in a few months. EBV parasitizes and immortalizes the lymphocytes. Infected lymphocytes continue to divide and their progeny—containing EBV—stay with us forever. There is a chance that a mutation will occur during each division of EBV-infected lymphocytes. Some mutations lead to cancerous growth of cells. Cancer derives from a cell line (clone) multiplying so rapidly that our immune system cannot destroy cells fast enough. As a result, the cells proliferate unchecked, spreading cancer throughout our body.

Meanwhile, EBV is working at another level to induce cancer by inserting part of its own gene into our human chromosomes, a process called integration. Integration may upset the natural balance of cellular reproduction. EBV-modified chromosomes might tell the cell to divide at two or three times its normal rate and not to respond to essential feedback signals that stop cells from ceaselessly dividing. Some host signals are enhanced, while others are jammed, causing the infected cells to behave in bizarre ways.

WHAT MONO VIRUS HAS TAUGHT US

Cancer from a kiss? Hardly. But EBV, the virus that causes "the kissing disease," is strongly linked to certain forms of human cancer. Does this mean we should curtail our kissing? Of course not. For most of us, mono is a mild or even asymptomatic illness. Only in the most unusual case does EBV provoke growth of tumor cells. To be afraid of acquiring cancer from EBV is like refusing to fly because the airplane might crash.

The cancer connection with EBV has provided us with important insights into how human viruses provoke cancer. The discovery by Dr. Hanto and colleagues that attacking the virus with an antiviral drug may avoid a cancerous state has exciting practical possibilities. EBV-cancer studies have supplied additional evidence of the importance of the immune surveillance system in destroying cancer cells. Young Jerry, for example, appeared to have his tumor under control until rejection therapy further weakened his immune system and gave EBV the upper hand.

As we have learned throughout *Herpes Diseases and Your Health,* herpesviruses produce a spectrum of illness ranging from inapparent infection to fatal encephalitis and even cancer. One-quarter to one-half of all EBV infections result in mono such as experienced by Kim and Charlie. In contrast, EBV's "big brother," cytomegalovirus (CMV), nearly always causes silent infections. Why then devote the next chapter to CMV, the least-known member of the herpesvirus clan? Because CMV can have profound medical consequences during pregnancy and after organ transplantation.

Cytomegalovirus:
Silent Cause of Birth Defects

"I'm not living next to that filthy little boy any more! We're moving out of this neighborhood," declared Adele Stevenson emphatically. So saying, she herded her husband, two-year-old son, nine-month-old daughter, and miscellaneous family treasures into the pickup and drove to her parents' farm 10 miles north of town. One day later, a realtor decorated the Stevenson's front lawn with his business address and phone number.

FOR SALE BY MIRROR LAKE REALTY. That sign was tangible proof of the power of misconceptions. It reminded me of a day long ago when the Health Department nailed a quarantine notice to our door after my sister broke out in measles. People were advised in writing to stay away from our house, and that made me feel unclean. The For Sale sign on the Stevenson's lawn was an ironic notice of contagion. Although Adam Pruitt, the "filthy little boy" next door, did have an infection, he was no risk to the woman who fled for fear of catching his virus.

Far from being filthy, the Pruitts were the most aseptic family in Mirror Lake, Minnesota. Jean Pruitt was a nurse. When she finally conceived after many childless years of marriage, she was both ecstatic and overwhelmed with responsibility. Jean devoured all the books she could find about infants and childrearing. One chapter of a pediatric text, which she read in the hospital library, particularly disturbed her. The chapter, entitled "Infections of the Newborn," stated that infants are more vulnerable to infections than adults because their immune systems are immature. Graphic descriptions of babies with specific infectious diseases followed. Jean first became concerned and then obsessed with the idea of protecting her baby from any and every infection. She prepared for her baby's arrival by scrubbing every room of the house weekly with disinfectant. She swabbed the designated nursery with double-strength solution. Jean compulsively washed her hands so many times a day that her knuckles became dry and cracked.

Jean went into labor right on schedule and delivered a vigorous six-pound boy, named Adam. He was normal in every respect, but Jean was not satisfied with the nurses' glowing reports. Any doctor who ventured on the maternity ward was interrogated at length about Adam's progress. Jean needed lots of reassurance! Just before discharge from Mirror Lake Community Hospital, Jean asked her physician, Dr. Bud Tucker, among other things, to send a sample of Adam's urine to the state virus laboratory.

"A consultant visited our hospital a few months ago, and I remember from his lecture that babies can be infected with certain viruses and have no symptoms at first," Jean said. "One virus with a funny name can be a big problem." Jean paused, then said hesitantly, "It's called . . . cytomegalovirus?"

"Ah yes, CMV," Dr. Tucker nodded. "My attitude, frankly, about medicine is that if you don't have a specific ailment, don't look for trouble. Adam is completely healthy. I see no need to do a urine culture."

But Jean persisted. "If Adam has any kind of infection whatsoever, I want to know it," she asserted. "I want to protect him and keep him as clean and healthy as possible."

"So what if we find CMV, Mrs. Pruitt?" The doctor was becoming impatient. "There's nothing we can do about it, you know."

"Dr. Tucker, that's short-sighted," Jean scolded. "Medical breakthroughs are being announced every time you turn on the news. Why, down in the Twin Cities three television stations have even hired reporters to cover medical news exclusively. I'll just bet there's been some important new information on CMV recently."

At this point, Bud Tucker had had enough. His operating schedule was full, and he had spent more time than he usually allocated for *routine* postpartum questions. Reluctantly, he wrote "urine specimen for CMV culture" on the discharge order sheet in Adam's chart.

Jean, true to her microbe phobia, would not permit the neighbors to touch Adam, for fear that they might be incubating strep throat or other dangerous bugs. Jean's husband, Herbert, thought that scrubbing the walls every week and shooing the neighbors away was ridiculous, but he did nothing to stop it. Herbert believed in minding his own business. Besides, he was never definite about anything.

Mirror Lake is a cozy rural town that prospers from a brisk summer tourist trade. Because most business is seasonal, the town has few year-round residents. Everyone is on a first-name basis, and gossip spreads faster than a prairie fire. Townsfolk began to murmur that something was wrong with the Pruitt baby. "Why not take Adam for a stroll outdoors? Why not let people hold him?" they wondered. As the weeks went by, Adam grew beautifully. He was smiling, and Jean was too, until a phone call came from Dr. Tucker's receptionist.

"Mrs. Pruitt, Adam's urine culture was positive for CMV. Dr. Tucker thinks you should come down to the clinic to have another sample checked."

Jean was beside herself; her worst fears had been realized. Her baby *had* been infected at birth with a horrible virus whose name she could hardly pronounce. Matters became worse when Dr. Tucker couldn't explain to Jean's satisfaction the medical consequences of Adam's positive urine culture.

The neighbors soon learned of Adam's CMV infection. Most felt sorry for the new parents and baby but didn't want to get directly involved. A few called to express sympathy or concern. But one in particular was worried—not about the baby but about herself. She was next-door neighbor Adele Stevenson, who had just read an article in a popular magazine about a new, deadly disease called AIDS. Adele remembered that AIDS, an acronym for Acquired Immunodeficiency Syndrome, was caused by CMV according to some researchers.

"AIDS is a new epidemic sweeping the country, and CMV is a strange new virus that causes AIDS," she reasoned aloud. "My lord, there's a baby living next door to us with CMV who might give us AIDS. We're getting out of here!"

Frederick Stevenson reassured his wife that Adam posed no risk to them because they hadn't seen him face to face.

"We don't know how AIDS is spread," she countered. "Maybe direct contact isn't necessary to catch this dreadful disease."

Adele's parents wanted her to think matters over before taking such a drastic step as moving. She consulted the minister, who reasoned with her to stay and be a good Samaritan to the Pruitt's. All arguments against moving were refuted in the end. Convinced she was saving her family from a fatal disease, Adele finally called the realtor.

The Mirror Lake episode is both comic and tragic. What could be more ridiculous than an adult running away from a baby she's never seen, for fear of an infection she knows next to nothing about? The tragedy: this story is based on a true incident, a sad consequence of a series of misconceptions that disrupted an entire family. The incident was brought to my attention by another Minnesota physician who sought my advice about explaining CMV contagion to his patients.

Before I tell you whether the Stevensons actually left their neighborhood forever, I want to point out five fallacies in Adele's reasoning.

- Cytomegalovirus (CMV) is not a new virus at all. Pathologists have known about it since the turn of the century.
- CMV is common in newborns. One percent of all babies born in the United States are infected. You can't distinguish them from their uninfected counterparts unless the doctor orders a urine test.
- CMV is very hard to catch. Transmission requires prolonged person-to-person contact.
- CMV poses only a minor risk to normal adults. A few adults develop an illness similar to infectious mononucleosis, but most have mild or asymptomatic CMV infections.
- CMV does not cause AIDS.

Adele and her family moved back home. Some said it was because high mortgage rates prevented the Stevensons from selling their house, while others blamed the perennial personality conflicts between Frederick and his in-laws. But the real reason was Dr. Bud Tucker's house call.

When word of Adele's hasty departure reached him, as it inevitably did the next day in that little town, Bud closed his office door and shook his head in disbelief.

"First, Jean overreacts to the possibility of CMV infection and *orders* me to send Adam's urine to the virus lab," he thought out loud. "Then her neighbors overreact even more to the way-out possibility that they will catch a fatal disease from a harmless infant. Unbelievable! I've got to set the record straight in a hurry."

That evening Dr. Tucker made an unscheduled visit to the farm where Adele was staying. He asked her to sit down with him alone in the sewing room.

"You and your family are at absolutely no risk of catching CMV from baby Adam unless you were to fondle him, kiss him, or handle his wet diapers without washing your hands," he told her. "Anyway, CMV is of no consequence to you, Adele, except if you catch it during pregnancy. Since you are not pregnant, we can forget about that problem. An association between CMV and AIDS has been made by some researchers, but from what I've read I don't believe that CMV is the cause of AIDS. Since you are a healthy woman and not a hemophiliac, the only conceivable way you could contract AIDS would be to use intravenous recreational drugs. And I am certain you are not a drug addict, Mrs. Stevenson."

Adele Stevenson doesn't like Dr. Tucker any more. "Why, the man practically accused me of being a junky," she has been overheard to exclaim. But his house call was effective in bringing her back to town and to reality.

Adam, now nearly two years old, is developing normally and no longer has CMV in his urine. A happy outcome like his is the rule for infants infected with CMV. But CMV is not always so benign: it's the leading cause of viral birth defects resulting in at least 3,000 brain-damaged infants in the United States every year. My experience with all five members of the herpes family has taught me that CMV is the most important herpesvirus for pregnant women, infants, and immunosuppressed patients.

ACQUISITION AND LATENCY
Carefully conducted prospective studies have shown that young adults pick up their first CMV infections at a rate of 2 to 3 percent per year. This is much lower than the 20 percent yearly acquisition rate of mono among college students. The rates of acquiring new CMV infections are strikingly similar for adults in Birmingham, Alabama, and Minneapolis, Minnesota, suggesting that CMV risk does not vary geographically.

Socioeconomic conditions do matter. Drs. Sergio Stagno and Charles Alford of the University of Alabama in Birmingham have shown that, as with herpes simplex and EBV, members of low income families catch CMV at an earlier age than those in middle- to high-income brackets. As with all the herpesviruses, person-to-person transmission appears to be facilitated by crowded living quarters.

CMV spreads more slowly and silently than the other herpesviruses. The majority of CMV infections are asymptomatic. Therefore, persons responsible for transmission don't know they are passing the virus around.

Most of us acquire CMV by mouth. CMV, like EBV, is found in saliva and can be contracted from kissing. CMV can spread to the infant during breast-feeding because CMV is present in mother's milk. Toddlers most likely acquire CMV through close contact with their peers. Day care centers have been implicated but not yet proven to be a source of CMV.

CMV is a true venereal disease just like herpes simplex. The virus has been grown from both male and female genital secretions. CMV can be acquired from fresh blood transfusions. Frozen red blood cells or freeze-dried blood products are not a source of CMV.

All herpesviruses have the capacity to remain dormant in the host for a time and then awaken. CMV is no exception. Most CMV infections result from reactivation of latent virus. The peculiar part of the CMV story is that we don't know where the virus resides during latency. Herpes simplex and varicella-zoster viruses hibernate in nerve cells; EBV sequesters itself in B-lymphocytes. CMV establishes latency neither in nerve cells nor in lymphocytes.

The reservoir for CMV may be the macrophage, a scavenger cell that migrates throughout our bloodstream and tissues searching for foreign invaders. When the macrophage encounters enemies, it "processes" them by changing their outside structure, making them targets for the immune artillery of the lymphocytes. Perhaps when the macrophage is stressed or damaged, latent CMV revives and multiplies.

DIAGNOSIS

A century ago, CMV was thought to be an amoeba, a large protozoan parasite. In the 1920s, pathologists recognized that tissue changes due to CMV resembled those found in chickenpox and herpes simplex infections. From then on, CMV was correctly considered a virus. CMV was cultivated in the laboratory in the mid-1950s by Dr. Margaret Smith in St. Louis and a group of investigators at the National Institutes of Health headed by Dr. Wallace Rowe. Diagnostic tests rapidly were developed, and today virus laboratories can detect CMV in throat swabs, urine, blood specimens, and biopsy material. Sensitive methods to measure CMV antibodies in blood samples are readily available. Tissue sections can be examined microscopically for CMV because the virus produces unique cellular changes. An infected cell resembles the eye of an owl looking straight at you. The pupil of that owl's eye is composed of partial virions—many, many viral particles being assembled in the nucleus of the infected cell. CMV contains the largest amount of DNA of all the human herpesviruses. That's why we sometimes refer to CMV as the "big brother" of the herpes family.

CMV IN "NORMAL" ADULTS

Editors of medical journals draw a red pencil through the word normal, arguing that there is no such thing as a "normal" patient. But

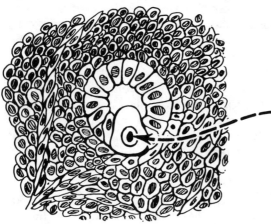

CMV being
formed inside
the nucleus
of a cell

Sketch of a microscopic section from a saliva gland infected with CMV. The virus has invaded a cell lining the central duct, causing the cell to enlarge and forming a mass within the nucleus that consists of many incomplete viral particles.

normal is a meaningful term to signify patients who are neither immunosuppressed nor chronically ill. For such individuals, CMV almost never causes more than a cold. Some adults develop a monolike CMV illness. Because CMV infections are so common, cases of anemia, arthritis, gastrointestinal ulcers, and encephalitis have been attributed to CMV. These complications of CMV in "normal" adults are so rare that we should not worry about them.

CMV IN PREGNANCY

Reactivation of CMV

CMV infections during pregnancy most commonly result from reactivation of virus acquired long ago. Many women have been infected with CMV before pregnancy, between 30 and 85 percent depending on socioeconomic status and geographical location. Silent recurrences of CMV are frequent in adults. Nearly 10 percent of pregnant women have CMV in their genital secretions near term.

When CMV reactivates during pregnancy, the baby may be infected before, during, or after birth. CMV is found in amniotic fluid, which cushions and bathes the fetus before birth. Since babies swallow amniotic fluid, they could drink CMV and become infected. CMV is present in the uterine cervix (the opening of the womb), and thus the baby can be infected during labor and delivery. CMV is also found in breast milk, which probably represents the most common source of CMV infection after birth.

Primary CMV Infection

If a woman acquires her first CMV infection during pregnancy, the virus enters the mother's circulating white blood cells and may traverse the placenta to infect the infant. Dr. Stagno and his Alabama coworkers studied 5,155 pregnant women to determine the effects of CMV on their offspring. They estimated that 1 percent acquired their very first CMV infection during pregnancy. Although 48 percent of their babies were infected, only five (14 percent) of 35 infants referred to the Alabama group were symptomatic. Just two of the five symptomatic babies were found to have brain damage. Therefore, the risk of having a sick baby due to your first CMV infection in pregnancy is 1.4 per thousand (0.01 × 0.14) and the risk of having a brain-damaged infant is 0.6 per thousand (0.01 × 0.06).

CMV IN INFANTS

CMV in infants is much more common than herpes simplex. One of every 100 babies born in the United States contracts CMV from the mother before, at, or shortly after delivery. Most of these infections, as I've just explained, result from reactivation of latent maternal CMV. Under these circumstances, the virus almost never produces obvious damage to the child. Such was Adam's case. About 10 percent of children infected by reactivation of maternal CMV eventually develop subtle hearing loss or changes in tooth enamel. Infants infected with CMV at birth should be checked by a pediatrician at least every six months during their first four years of life. Hearing loss, if detected, should be corrected quickly so that speech develops normally.

Infected infants do not rid themselves of CMV for a long time. Virus is present in the throat and urine for at least two years, but these babies are not very contagious. Nurses who care for CMV-infected infants do not acquire CMV at a faster rate than their nonmedical contemporaries, recent studies have shown. Therefore, babies do not readily transmit CMV to hospital personnel even though such infants receive intimate, long-term intensive care. The nurse studies teach us that you can effectively protect yourself from catching CMV by washing your hands after handling an infected child or the wet diapers.

CMV infections that attack the fetus before birth are called congenital. Congenital CMV almost always results from primary maternal infection. If CMV crosses the placenta from mother to baby, virus can damage developing fetal organs. These include the brain, heart, intestinal tract, muscles, and bones. CMV is the most devastating to the brain because if neurons are destroyed, they do not regenerate. Few infants with congenital CMV are symptomatic at birth, and therefore pediatricians frequently do not suspect CMV until follow-up examination reveals delayed development.

QUESTIONS FROM CONCERNED PARENTS

These questions from my patients represent common concerns about CMV in pregnant women and their offspring.

Q. I babysit occasionally for a neighbor who recently learned that her baby daughter has CMV. I've just discovered I'm pregnant. What should I do?

A. Not to worry. Washing your hands after close contact with a baby who has CMV will prevent you from catching the virus. Even if you didn't wash your hands, transmission of CMV requires close and prolonged contact. Occasional babysitting will not result in your catching CMV from the child.

Q. I am eight weeks pregnant. Are there any activities that I should avoid to protect myself from CMV?

A. Essentially none. I do advise pregnant women not to kiss or have sexual relations with a person who has had an infectious mononucleosis-like illness within the past three months. CMV sometimes produces mono symptoms in adults, and CMV is transmitted by saliva and genital secretions. Mono virus, EBV, has been implicated as a rare cause of birth defects, and pregnant women would not want to pick up EBV either.

Q. Should my doctor draw a blood sample to find out if I am immune to CMV before I become pregnant?

A. At present this is the most difficult question concerning CMV for young women. One thing is certain—if you are contemplating pregnancy and decide you want to be tested, have the blood drawn *before* you conceive. Antibodies develop within seven to 10 days after CMV infects you. Finding antibodies, for example, during the second trimester of pregnancy could be the result of a first infection during pregnancy *or* an infection before pregnancy. A first infection during pregnancy is of much greater consequence than a CMV infection long ago. If the test is done before you conceive and you have CMV antibodies, your baby will not develop the primary form of CMV infection. That's good, but we cannot guarantee that your child won't become infected from reactivation of your old CMV. If he or she catches the virus from you, your antibodies will modify the severity of infection. However, some babies born to "immune" mothers eventually develop hearing loss. Thus CMV immunity is a relative rather than an absolute condition.

Women who lack CMV antibody sometimes become overly concerned about the dangers of infection in their infants. If you do not have CMV antibodies during pregnancy, the most important thing to remember is that CMV is hard to catch. Wash your hands after handling infants, diapers, or patients with suspected CMV infections, and avoid kissing friends on the lips.

Q. My baby boy is completely healthy, but I am concerned about CMV. Should I have his urine tested for CMV?

A. No. I agree with Dr. Bud Tucker. Babies should be tested for CMV only if your doctor has reason to suspect a CMV infection. Testing every baby is just too expensive. One of 100 infants has CMV in the urine, and one of 10 CMV-infected babies will develop a hearing deficit. The average viral culture charge is $35. If the urine of every baby were cultured, the cost per hearing-impaired child would be $35,000. Subtle clinical findings, which doctors call "soft" signs, observed during routine checkups will tip off your physician or nurse practitioner to look for CMV.

Q. Is there future hope for completely preventing CMV infections?

A. Yes. A CMV vaccine has been developed by Dr. Stanley Plotkin and colleagues at Children's Hospital of Philadelphia. This vaccine is presently being tested in patients awaiting kidney transplants. If found safe and effective for them, CMV vaccine may be approved for use in "normal" susceptible women. See the discussion of CMV vaccine later in this chapter.

Q. My eight-year-old son Joshua has CMV. Because he is hearing-impaired, he attends a special school. Recently, parents of other pupils have expressed concern for their children. Can they get CMV from Joshua?

A. Joshua, and children like him, should not be excluded from school because they have CMV. It is highly unlikely that Joshua would infect anyone, and even if another child picked up CMV, the virus would cause few or no symptoms. Personnel can protect themselves by washing their hands if they have hands-on contact with your child.

Q. If breast milk contains CMV, wouldn't it be better to bottle-feed my baby?

A. No. Breast milk is probably our most natural source of CMV. In a sense, CMV in breast milk immunizes children. In my opinion, after babies are born they do not have any greater problems with CMV than adults. It is far better for a girl to get CMV for the first time during childhood than during pregnancy.

CMV AFTER ORGAN TRANSPLANTATION

More than 6,000 Americans receive organ transplants in the United States every year. About half of them will develop a CMV infection within a few weeks after surgery. Here is the story of one patient who did.

Ted: Balanced on a Tightrope

Ted is a high-powered executive at a large midwestern corporation. His illness, he told me, started shortly after a gala fortieth-birthday celebration in his honor. He became very thirsty, which he attributed to eating lots of potato chips at the party. He also noticed that he was urinating much more than usual. When these symptoms didn't improve after more than a week, he consulted his internist, whom he had not seen for several years because he considered himself to be in excellent health.

Nothing was apparent on physical examination, but blood tests revealed that Ted's kidney function was poor. A number of diagnostic procedures followed, including a biopsy of one of his kidneys. The results were shocking: Ted was suffering from irreversible kidney failure – cause unknown. He had two alternatives: chronic hemodialysis (a mechanical method of removing toxic substances from the bloodstream) or kidney transplantation. Ted's job and life style were not suited to spending six hours a week in a hemodialysis unit, so he opted for renal transplantation. His internist eventually referred him to the University of Minnesota.

I first met Ted during his pretransplant workup. My research group was conducting an experimental CMV vaccine program in collaboration with the transplant surgeons. In the normal course of events, my chief nurse would explain the pros and cons of CMV vaccine. Patients who consented were enrolled in the program and assigned to vaccine or placebo. For some reason, the nurse's explanation did not satisfy Ted and he asked to see me.

Ted appeared cocky and abrasive, but I quickly diagnosed this as a defense mechanism. Like so many transplant candidates, Ted was genuinely frightened. The process of kidney transplantation is still relatively new and there is much to learn about preventing rejection of the organ (our natural immune response to the foreign, transplanted kidney) and infection. Patients must digest a mountain of literature about the surgery and its consequences. Ted was used to being the boss. His way of coping with this avalanche of events was to bully the medical staff.

I explained the CMV vaccine trial to Ted, informing him that in our hospital about half the patients develop CMV infection after transplantation. Most CMV infections are mild, but for about a third of the patients the illness prolongs hospitalization. Some CMV infections even result in loss of the kidney. I told Ted that in order to determine if the vaccine works, some patients are vaccinated and some are given a placebo, which in this study is the fluid used to reconstitute the vaccine. Neither he nor I would know what he received so that results could in no way be biased.

Ted challenged me with difficult questions about the complications of immunization and its implications for transplantation. Finally satisfied with my answers, he agreed to participate in the trial.

Several months later, at age 41, Ted received a kidney from his older brother. The surgery went smoothly, his new kidney functioned almost immediately, and he was discharged after two weeks.

All went well for a month. Ted was back on the job part-time. Then one night he woke up with a shaking chill. The next morning his wife noticed that the bedsheets were soaking wet, and his temperature was 102 degrees Fahrenheit. She phoned the transplant office and was instructed to bring Ted to the clinic as soon as possible. Doctors found no evidence of infection anywhere in Ted's body. Fever persisted, however, and several days later Ted was admitted to the Transplant Service at University Hospitals. Despite extensive diagnostic tests, the cause of his fever remained obscure. Biopsy of his transplanted kidney did not reveal rejection, which can cause fever after transplantation.

At the beginning of his third week in the hospital, Ted developed a cough. His legs ached, and he had trouble walking. Chest X rays revealed whitish, fluffy areas throughout both lungs. After inspecting the X ray films, an intern wrote in Ted's chart "impression—probable cytomegalovirus pneumonia."

Surgeons explained to Ted that the most important way to combat his presumed CMV infection was to decrease his immunosuppressive drugs. "We're walking a tightrope," they told him, "because these drugs keep your newly transplanted kidney from being rejected. Yet, our immune system is a vital defense against CMV. By decreasing your immunosuppression, we give the immune defenses a better chance."

After tapering Ted's doses of azathioprine and prednisone—the very drugs that protected his transplanted organ—surgeons watched anxiously as his kidney function deteriorated. Would Ted fend off the CMV infection before his new kidney was destroyed by rejection?

I was consulted about Ted a second time. I explained to him that our virus laboratory still had not confirmed his diagnosis because CMV grows very, very slowly. On the positive side, I was able to tell him that the vast majority of kidney transplant patients with CMV infections, even those with pneumonia, recover.

Several days later, a urine sample collected from Ted the day before hospitalization was positive for CMV and soon a blood culture grew CMV too. The diagnosis of CMV infection was established. During the fourth week of illness Ted's fever showed signs of breaking, but his cough had worsened and his legs remained weak. His white blood cell count was dangerously low, indicating limited ability to fight any infection. By the fifth week, Ted was improving at last. His fever was gone. His eyes regained their devilish spark, and he began to badger nurses and doctors about the whys and wherefores of their seemingly incessant rounds. Previously bedridden except for very short periods, he could now walk down the hall wheeling his intravenous apparatus alongside. When I overheard Ted heckling the chief transplant surgeon, I knew that he was going to recover fully.

Ted left the hospital after six weeks. CMV had significantly complicated his transplantation but left no permanent scars. We all were relieved to see him walk off the ward arm-in-arm with his wife. He was fortunate—10 percent of kidney transplant patients who develop CMV pneumonia never leave intensive care.

We have not yet opened the sealed envelopes to find out whether Ted received CMV vaccine or placebo because our vaccine tests are not finished. One thing is obvious as our trial draws to a close: CMV vaccine is not perfect. There is still no ideal way to prevent CMV infections after transplantation. But this vaccine may be an important first step.

What CMV Means to Transplant Patients: An Analogy

Years ago in an editorial for the *Archives of Internal Medicine*, I nicknamed CMV "the Troll of Transplantation." The behavior of CMV after kidney transplantation reminded me of a children's story, "The Three Billy Goats Gruff." The billy goats, you may recall, wanted to cross over a river to get to greener pastures. A troll lay in wait under the bridge. As the billy goats stepped onto the wooden bridge one by one, the troll emerged and threatened to gobble them up. After months or years on hemodialysis, the transplant patient finally receives a new kidney. Kidney function returns, and the patient regains appetite and vigor. The transplant recipient figuratively crosses over the bridge from chronic disease to good health. Just as that halcyon period begins, CMV jumps out from its hiding place and threatens the patient's newfound well-being.

Conclusions from the Kidney Transplant Experience

Drs. Richard Simmons and John Najarian discovered more than a decade ago at the University of Minnesota that CMV is the primary cause of infection after kidney transplantation. The CMV-transplant problem was so great that it fostered the growth of virology services now available for *all* our patients. What has been learned about CMV from kidney transplant patients during this time?

• CMV infections in immunosuppressed patients most often are due to reactivation of CMV acquired long before transplantation. These infections are milder on the whole than CMV infections contracted for the first time at transplantation.

• If patients develop their first CMV infection during transplantation, virus most likely comes from the donated organ or from blood transfusions.

• CMV infections tend to occur two weeks to two months after kidney transplantation. Most patients have fever—nothing else. Some develop pneumonia and muscle weakness, as Ted did. A few suffer from intestinal ulcers, liver inflammation, and encephalitis. Today doctors know when to look for CMV infection, how to recognize it, and how to judiciously decrease immunosuppression so that the patient can combat his or her infection.

• Long-term surveillance studies show that the risk of catching CMV from another transplant patient or from hospital personnel is nil. Patients are unlikely to transmit CMV to anyone except their spouses. Therefore, elaborate isolation measures for patients are unnecessary.

• Surveys of CMV infections after kidney transplantation have led to similar investigations in other immunosuppressed patients with identical results: CMV is a very common and significant infection for heart, liver, and bone marrow transplant recipients and cancer patients.

• Children born to kidney transplant patients have not sustained congenital CMV infections. Although numbers are still too small to draw absolute conclusions, these babies seem to be protected against CMV despite their mother's depressed immunity.

• Preliminary results from Philadelphia and Minneapolis suggest that CMV vaccine cannot prevent all CMV infections but lessens their severity.

• Treatment of CMV may be within our grasp. The drug acyclovir was beneficial in a small study conducted at the University of Minnesota (see chapter 9). A derivative of acyclovir has been found to be 10 times more effective than the parent drug against CMV in laboratory tests. Finally, scientists at the Sloane-Kettering Institute for Cancer Research in New York City have developed a new series of compounds that show great promise against CMV.

THE AIDS CONNECTION

AIDS, an acronym for Acquired Immunodeficiency Syndrome, *is* a new disease, but AIDS is not sweeping the country. AIDS strikes almost exclusively three population groups: male homosexuals, users of intravenous recreational drugs, and hemophiliacs. Of the more than 3,000 cases meeting the CDC criteria for AIDS at the end of 1983, nearly 90 percent fit into one of these three groups. Our best evidence suggests that AIDS is either sexually transmitted or acquired through injections of blood and blood products.

Because the cause of AIDS has not been discovered, definition of the disease remains imprecise. AIDS is best described as an unexplained, rather abrupt loss of normal immune function. The loss of immunity is signaled by development of one of eight specific disease states that would not ordinarily be found in otherwise healthy young adults. These diseases fit the category of either opportunistic infections—infections that occur only in immunologically crippled patients—or cancers. AIDS often begins as a unique cancer, called Kaposi's sarcoma after the Austrian dermatologist who first described the tumor in 1872. Kaposi's sarcoma causes red bumps on the skin that are very characteristic of the condition. Symptoms common in AIDS patients are fevers of unknown cause, loss of weight, weakness, pneumonia, diarrhea, and progressive deterioration of brain function.

Despite the carping of a House subcommittee and some special interest groups, an impressive national campaign has been mounted to understand the cause of AIDS and devise methods of prevention or treatment. The Department of Health and Human Services allocated $48.2 million in 1984 alone to combat AIDS, according to spokeswoman Shirley Barth.

Several scientists were enthusiastic about early reports linking CMV to AIDS. The strongest argument favoring a CMV etiology is that most AIDS patients have CMV antibody. However, this merely tells us that AIDS patients have been infected with CMV sometime in their lives, not that CMV causes AIDS. A number of factors militate against CMV as the cause. The most compelling is that some AIDS patients lack CMV antibody. Another factor concerns the way hemophiliacs contract AIDS. Hemophiliacs face an increased risk for AIDS, presumably because the AIDS agent is in the blood products they receive to control bleeding. But since CMV does not survive freezing or drying—processes used in the preparation of blood products for hemophiliacs—the AIDS agent must be something other than CMV.

AIDS is caused by a virus, current research indictates, probably in the same family as the human T-cell leukemia virus discovered in 1980 and classified as a retrovirus. In support of this view, studies of an AIDS-like disease in rhesus monkeys have implicated a blood-borne simian retrovirus as the culprit. Although not the cause of AIDS, CMV may increase the patient's susceptibility to AIDS because CMV by itself is immunosuppressive. Perhaps CMV, acquired by the patient during the pre-AIDS period, leads to an immunosuppressive state so profound that another virus or microbial agent normally incapable of producing disease gains a foothold, multiplies, and the syndrome now recognized as AIDS develops.

CMV is certainly a problem for patients after they develop AIDS. AIDS patients are severely immunosuppressed. Their immunosuppression is graver than that of any organ transplant patient. CMV threatens AIDS victims just as it does organ transplant patients. Methods for prevention and treatment of CMV infections now being tested in transplant patients may help AIDS sufferers as well. AIDS patients need all the help they can get because the majority eventually die of their disease. This lethal aspect of AIDS frightened Adele Stevenson so much that she panicked and ran away from a harmless infant before learning the facts.

CMV IN PERSPECTIVE

Two decades ago, at least 30,000 newborns in the United States suffered major birth defects due to rubella virus. Shortly after that national disaster, rubella vaccine was developed and tested successfully in children. By 1970, rubella immunization became routine practice in the United States. Today, because 95 percent of children entering elementary school have received rubella vaccine, congenital rubella has all but disappeared. With the elimination of congenital rubella, CMV now ranks as the number-one viral cause of birth defects, accounting for approximately 3,000 damaged babies yearly in the United States. Birth defects are both a tragedy for the involved family and a chronic drain on society's health dollar. We must be alert for medical research developments concerning CMV. As soon as an acceptable method of CMV prevention—most likely a vaccine—becomes available, I urge you and your family to make use of it. If CMV is ever to be eliminated as a cause of birth defects, awareness of the problem must begin now so that citizens are not apathetic. A major reason for failure of some vaccination campaigns in the past has been public indifference.

CMV infects most children without harming them but unpredictably injures a few. Had Adam Pruitt been my patient, I would have told his mother, Jean, just what Dr. Bud Tucker said: "A positive CMV culture from baby Adam probably means nothing. Most CMV-infected babies never have problems. On the other hand, Adam eventually could develop hearing loss. To diagnose and correct that, he needs to see his pediatrician every six months." Based on current medical studies, neither Bud nor I could give Jean an exact prognosis.

We have fewer answers than we would like about CMV. However, our central theme—knowledge is power—still holds. Armed with the information you now have, you can help dispel misconceptions about CMV that crop up in your community. Adele Stevenson is not alone in her unfounded fear of CMV. Schools inappropriately have expelled CMV-infected pupils, not realizing that CMV is of little consequence for normal children and adults. Pregnant personnel are at some risk, but can completely protect themselves by washing their hands after contact with an infected child.

What is being done to solve the CMV problem for pregnant women and immunosuppressed patients? At the molecular level, CMV is drawing rapt attention from virologists. In many laboratories across the country, CMV's DNA—its heritable information—is being chewed up into recognizable fractions by special bacterial enzymes. Components of CMV's outside coat are being separated, purified, and analyzed. Our goals are twofold: to find exactly where CMV is most vulnerable to biochemical attack; and to determine which part of the virus, if used as a vaccine, will induce long-lasting immunity without producing side effects.

Effective Therapies for Herpes Diseases

Recent advances in treatment of herpesvirus infections are astounding. Remember Mike Peterson (chapter 5), the 10-year-old leukemic child who died of chickenpox? His death could have been averted today. Children like Mike, with severely damaged immune systems, not only are surviving their chickenpox but are walking out of the hospital with no aftereffects, thanks to the exciting advances in antiviral therapy.

To begin this fast-moving medical saga, let's listen to one of my patients who was among the first to receive the antiviral drug acyclovir during clinical tests. The following interview was conducted in Minneapolis for an educational film now being shown to help doctors treat herpes infections.

MONICA'S MOVIE INTERVIEW

Monica: I was very down when doctors told me I had cancer. I had a sore on my cheek that didn't heal, so I went to have a physical and they diagnosed me at that time as having lymphoma. I was told that cancer drugs could make my illness go away for a time and maybe never return. The drugs were horrible. I was sick to my stomach, I vomited, my hair fell out, but finally my cancer was going away—going into remission. I became less depressed. I started calling friends on the telephone. I was even getting an appetite for hospital food. Just when I was perking up, I developed a fever, and my mouth and chin became sore. The doctors told me I had herpes.

Interviewer: Did you know what *herpes* meant?

Monica: Herpes is a virus, right? I thought herpes only caused cold sores, annoying little things that come out on your face sometimes when you are sick from another virus. I'm 50, and I've had cold sores on and off for most of my adult life. They were an annoyance, nothing more. So what herpes meant was confusing to me. This wasn't cold sores; this was hell. It was painful to eat, and, consequently, I had to have my food blended. When people would call me on the telephone, I would have to tell them they had to talk instead of me because it did hurt. I don't like to remember the pain of it.

Interviewer: Did the doctors do anything to help your herpes?

Monica: Yes. My cancer doctor told me there was nothing proven to work against herpes but that Dr. Balfour was involved in testing a new drug. He asked if I would be interested. I told him I was.

Interviewer: Did the thought of taking an experimental drug make you anxious?

Monica: Oh goodness, no. I have been used to this with all the different experimental programs they have for cancer patients. This was just another new drug to me. Besides, my pain was so bad that I was willing to try anything.

Interviewer: What happened next?

Monica: Dr. Balfour's team explained to me that this was a study to learn if the drug acyclovir really worked. To find out, only some of the patients would get acyclovir injections into their veins; others would just get the sugar water in which acyclovir was mixed. They explained that neither they nor I would know what I had been given until the trial was over. They told me I had a 50 percent chance of getting drug and a 50 percent chance of getting just the I.V. fluid. I felt that half a chance was better than no chance at all so I signed the papers and told them to get on with it.

Interviewer: Did the drug help you?

Monica: Well, you see, I didn't know for some time whether I'd been given the drug or not. All I can tell you is that for the first two days the pain was excruciating. I was depressed, I didn't want to talk to my friends, I couldn't talk to my friends. I cried a lot. When I woke up on the third day, the burning was better. I sipped some liquids through a straw, but still I couldn't eat any solid food. The next day I was definitely better, and I was able to eat jello and soft things like that. By the end of this study, which lasted a week, I knew that I was on the way to getting better. My mouth didn't completely heal for several weeks, but I could carry on conversations and became more cheerful. As you can see [pointing to her chin], when all the sores healed they left me with some scarring. It has been two years since that herpes infection, and I have not had a recurrence.

Interviewer: What was your reaction when the research nurse called you after the study was finished and said that you had received acyclovir?

Monica: I wasn't surprised. I knew, I just knew something was going on when I was getting those I.V.s. It was more than just imagination; something was making me better.

Interviewer: Some people find it hard to believe that cold sores can be an important medical problem. This is even true for doctors. In this movie we're making for doctors, we are trying to help them realize the problems that herpes can cause for patients such as yourself who have cancer. Can you think of anything to say to doctors that might be helpful?

Monica: Tell them that the pain can be hard to live with. I have no pain now, but some day my cancer might come back and I'll have to be hospitalized for more cancer treatments. I can live with that, my cancer I mean, but I am afraid of the herpes. I am more afraid of herpes than the cancer treatments.

Comment: Severe oral herpes like Monica's occurs only in cancer patients and others who are immunosuppressed. Fortunately, the success of antiviral drugs is not limited to difficult, complicated cases like hers. Breakthroughs in treatment of the common diseases due to herpes simplex and varicella-zoster virus have been achieved. Here is an analysis, disease by disease, of the key advances made possible by careful clinical trials.

SEVEN HERPESVIRUS DISEASES THAT CAN BE TREATED

Genital Herpes

Until 1982 physicians could offer their patients no medically proven treatment for genital herpes. Of course, quack cures and home remedies abounded—everything from skin dyes to vitamin pills—but none was supported by objective, scientific data.

Acyclovir Ointment. In March 1982, the federal Food and Drug Administration licensed acyclovir ointment after four years of evaluation in patients. The FDA commissioner called the new prescription ointment "a step forward" in treatment. He cautioned, however, that acyclovir "is not a cure for herpesvirus infections." That caveat was echoed by several other scientists.

As a result, some of you with genital herpes read or were told that acyclovir can't help you. Why? A surprising thing happened after licensure of acyclovir ointment, something almost unprecedented in the history of drug research. When acyclovir ointment actually became available by prescription, no scientific reports about its use had yet been published in the professional medical literature. Physicians had nothing to read to satisfy themselves, as they must do, that a drug is safe and beneficial for their patients. Doctors lacked reliable sources for answers to critical questions about whom to treat, how long to treat, and when to treat the patients again. This information vacuum permitted a few researchers who were critical of acyclovir to have their say, and several decried use of acyclovir ointment for a practical and a theoretical reason. One skeptic even commented in the editorial column of the *New England Journal of Medicine*, "The patient can more wisely spend the $16 to $24 price of a 15-g tube of ointment on something else."

The practical concern was valid. Acyclovir ointment can only be used to treat superficial infections because it works at or near the site of application. Our protective layer of skin cells allows just a small amount of drug to enter the bloodstream. Viral particles living deep inside the body escape unharmed because the virus-fighting drug never reaches them.

Some scientists theorized that widespread use of acyclovir ointment would lead to rapid emergence of resistant viruses—herpes strains that could multiply merrily in the presence of acyclovir. This hypothesis is incorrect; viral resistance to acyclovir is not a problem. Yet, the good news about acyclovir temporarily was lost in controversy.

Shortly after licensure of topical acyclovir, Dr. Lawrence Corey published a study in the *New England Journal of Medicine*. Corey and colleagues at the University of Washington clearly demonstrated the antiviral potency of acyclovir in patients with first episodes of genital herpes. To prove effectiveness of acyclovir, all the volunteers received look-alike tubes, half containing acyclovir, half containing placebo (a harmless substance of no therapeutic value). Neither the scientists nor the patients knew which tube was which. The volunteers were examined nearly every day. Sores were observed for healing, then cultured to learn if herpes was still alive. When the study was completed, eureka! Virus was killed on average within three days in patients who used acyclovir ointment, but herpes was alive in the sores for nearly seven days in the placebo group. After death of the offending organisms, healing proceeded apace. Herpes sores healed two days faster in the acyclovir-treated patients than in the placebo group.

Based on Corey's publication and several other studies, I concluded that acyclovir ointment benefits all patients with external genital herpes sores because: duration of infection is shortened, decreasing the likelihood of spreading genital herpes; and healing is accelerated, helping the patient feel better and resume sexual activity sooner.

Acyclovir ointment should not be applied inside the mouth or in the internal genital tract, a definite limitation. You might be discouraged by that and ask, "Is ointment the only way acyclovir can be given?" Absolutely not.

Acyclovir Injections and Capsules. Acyclovir comes in several other forms including intravenous injections and capsules, both of which are more effective than acyclovir ointment. Like antibiotics, acyclovir is most powerful when injected into a vein. Acutely ill patients willing to be hospitalized clearly benefit from intravenous injections of acyclovir. In the test studies, acyclovir-treated patients with first attacks of genital herpes experienced only three days of pain, compared with seven days for those receiving placebo. In the typical patient, intravenous acyclovir cuts the duration of genital herpes in half.

What if you're not sick enough to warrant injections by vein? The average patient doesn't need an intravenous drug. In fact, most would probably refuse it. Here comes the best news yet—acyclovir capsules taken by mouth are effective treatment for initial episodes of genital herpes. When the pills become available, they will be the treatment of choice.

Acyclovir capsules are also effective in managing recurrent genital herpes. A study completed in 1983 by Corey's Seattle-based research group found that recurrences of genital herpes can be stalled by taking acyclovir capsules for several months. Such use of acyclovir is termed suppressive therapy. Scientists are actively investigating the safety of long-term acyclovir suppressive therapy in patients with frequent recurrences.

Dr. Richard Reichman of the University of Rochester Medical Center, New York, wrote in the April 27, 1984, issue of the *Journal of the American Medical Association* that acyclovir capsules provided a significant *treatment* benefit in a placebo-controlled study of more than 100 patients with active recurrent genital herpes.

Treatment versus Cure. You might have read that acyclovir cannot cure genital herpes. When the ointment was approved, even the FDA commissioner commented that he did not consider the drug a cure-all. The scientific community changes its mind slowly, but recent clinical evidence indicates acyclovir may cure some patients with genital herpes after all. UCLA's Dr. Yvonne Bryson reported surprising results in Vienna at an international medical meeting held during September 1983. Her volunteers were patients with first episodes of genital herpes. Half of them received acyclovir capsules, while half swallowed placebo pills. The acyclovir-treated patients showed marked clinical improvement of their acute infection, not surprising in view of Corey's results with acyclovir ointment. During the next six months, acyclovir-treated patients experienced the same number of recurrences as those given placebo, also not surprising. After that, to our astonishment, acyclovir patients endured significantly fewer recurrences than the placebo subjects!

Why did the virus seem to melt away after six months? Let's suppose that virions penetrated 500 nerve cell bodies in the sacral ganglia during a first episode of genital herpes. Let's assume a recurrence represents reactivation of virions inside a single neuron. The neuron is destroyed when virions awaken, multiply, and migrate down the nerve fibers to create a new genital herpes infection. If recurrences happen once a month, that patient theoretically could look forward to 500 recurrences spanning 500 months. Some of those virions would outsleep Rip Van Winkle!

If the patient receives acyclovir during the first episode of genital herpes, many virions are killed by the drug before they can reach the sacral ganglia. Perhaps only enough virions escape to infect a half-dozen neurons. If the patient experiences monthly recurrences, all the infected neurons would be destroyed after six months, leaving no more latent virus inside the body to perpetuate recurrences. In a real sense, the patient is cured of genital herpes.

Is acyclovir the only hope for genital herpes victims? Right now acyclovir is the only drug available. Several drugs potentially useful against genital herpes are being tested in patients. But more time is needed to prove that these drugs are safe, effective, and worthy of FDA approval. The new drugs include arildone, undergoing clinical trials in the United States, and foscarnet, which is being studied in Europe. Ribavirin tablets appeared to reduce the severity and duration of pain in recurrent genital herpes in a study of California patients. Interferon is being tested in patients with recurrent genital herpes. Although some encouraging preliminary results have been reported, these must be confirmed by more extensive clinical investigation.

Herpes of the Mouth, Lips, and Skin

Cold Sores in "Normal" Adults. English researchers reported that acyclovir cream accelerated healing in 49 British Petroleum employees with recurrent oral herpes. Their results were published in the May 28, 1983, issue of the *British Medical Journal*. Dr. Spotswood Spruance of the University of Utah, on the other hand, reported significantly swifter killing of herpes in 208 patients, who had used acyclovir ointment, but lip lesions did not heal faster as a result of this therapy.

Will acyclovir or another antiviral drug prove worthwhile for recurrent cold sores? Most patients have a premonition that herpes is recurring before blisters erupt. For oral and genital herpes, the prodrome is usually a tingling at the exact site where blisters are coming. Ointment applied as soon as tingling starts may result in a shorter period of infection or prevent cold sores from erupting at all. A 1983 study at London's Eastman Dental Hospital confirmed the efficacy of this approach, called expectant therapy, among 31 patients who applied acyclovir ointment as soon as they experienced the prodrome. The researchers concluded, "Acyclovir ointment is well tolerated and appears to modify the course of severe recurrent herpes labialis when therapy is initiated by the patient during the prodrome."

Acyclovir pills should be more useful than ointment for oral herpes because the drug enters the bloodstream and could destroy virions migrating down the nerve pathways before they reach the skin.

Infections in Immunosuppressed Patients. Herpes infections in immunosuppressed patients are more troublesome, lasting longer, causing more pain, and spreading more widely. Success of intravenous acyclovir against herpes simplex infections was reported by our Minnesota group in the June 1981 edition of the international medical journal, *Lancet*. The immune systems of our patients were weakened by cancer or organ transplantation before their herpes infections erupted. The majority of the patients had severe oral herpes. Monica was one of 24 Minnesota patients who helped prove that acyclovir reduces pain and kills the virus. Our patients were part of a group of 97 treated at 11 medical centers in North America. The information gathered from this collaborative study established that acyclovir was safe and effective against herpes infections of the skin and mucous membranes in immunosuppressed patients. The FDA has licensed intravenous acyclovir for this purpose.

Herpes in the Eye
Four antiviral drugs are very effective against herpes in the eye (herpes keratitis). These are idoxuridine, trifluorothymidine, vidarabine, and acyclovir. Acyclovir eye ointment is not yet FDA-approved. Herpetic eye infections should always be managed by an ophthalmologist because herpes keratitis frequently recurs and eye surgery occasionally is needed to preserve sight.

Herpes Encephalitis
Herpes encephalitis has tragic consequences for its victims. More than half will die, and those who survive often are left with permanently damaged nervous systems. Thanks to the original work of Dr. Richard Whitley in Birmingham, Alabama, vidarabine was found to be an effective treatment for herpes encephalitis. Just a year after a landmark article published by Dr. Whitley and his colleagues in the *New England Journal of Medicine* in 1977, vidarabine was licensed by the FDA for treatment of herpes encephalitis. Vidarabine has cut mortality of herpes encephalitis nearly in half: from 70 to 38 percent. Unfortunately, brain damage was common among drug-treated survivors. The search to improve quality of life for survivors of herpes encephalitis continues.

Neonatal Herpes
Herpes in the newborn is just as severe as herpes encephalitis. Pioneering studies by Dr. André Nahmias of Emory University in Atlanta clearly defined the importance of this entity in the 1960s. Vidarabine has benefited infants with neonatal herpes, but so far results have been discouragingly similar to those reported for herpes encepha-

litis. More vidarabine-treated babies survived than placebo recipients, but there was evidence of permanent nervous-system damage in many of the survivors. New studies employing either higher doses of vidarabine or acyclovir are under way. See Jeremy's story at the end of this chapter.

Chickenpox

Chickenpox is one of the most dreaded infections at any medical center. Just a few years ago, when leukemic children such as Mike Peterson developed chickenpox, we had no treatment to offer them. We prayed that their immune systems would fight off the virus before it was too late. We breathed for them with mechanical ventilators and maintained their blood pressure with drugs. But we lost the battle to save their lives when the virus invaded the lungs, the central nervous system, or the intestines. Today, however, we know that both vidarabine and acyclovir are potentially lifesaving for these patients.

The average child with chickenpox does not need antiviral drugs, but some do experience complications such as skin infections and joint inflammation. Acyclovir pills may become acceptable treatment for such complications in the near future until chickenpox vaccine wipes out the disease entirely.

Shingles

In 1978, Dr. Thomas Merigan's team at Stanford University, Palo Alto, California, reported that interferon arrested the spread of shingles if given no later than three days after immunosuppressed adults developed the rash. Dr. Richard Whitley's group reported in the *New England Journal of Medicine* (1977 and 1982) that early vidarabine treatment accelerated healing, decreased pain, and prevented complications of shingles in immunosuppressed patients. My colleagues and I reported in the *New England Journal of Medicine* in June 1983 that intravenous acyclovir halted progression of shingles in immunosuppressed patients, even when given to patients whose rash was two weeks old. Shingles, once a major scourge for cancer and organ transplant patients, has come under the control of antiviral drugs.

What about normal patients who suffer from shingles? Shingles can be very painful and the pain so unrelenting that patients such as Lucille (see chapter 6) no longer can work. Acyclovir reduces pain and hastens skin healing if given by vein within three days of onset of rash. There are hints that the chronic pain of shingles (postherpetic neuralgia) might be prevented if acyclovir or vidarabine is given shortly after the rash appears. Acyclovir capsules are being studied for shingles treatment because intravenous injections, although clearly effective, are awkward. Intravenous treatment involves repeated trips to doctors' offices or emergency rooms, or actual hospitalization.

Can postherpetic neuralgia be treated? That possibility is being explored at the University of Minnesota using two months of acyclovir in both intravenous and oral forms. If the pain is due to multiplication of varicella-zoster virus within the nerve, antiviral drugs might be useful. On the other hand, if the pain is the result of permanent damage to nerve endings, such drugs won't work.

HERPESVIRUS DISEASES ELUDING TREATMENT

Infectious Mononucleosis

Young adults, especially college students, frequently seek medical help for infectious mononucleosis. They may even require hospitalization for a week or more. In a study of bedridden mono patients, intravenous acyclovir provided some improvement, such as regaining the weight lost during the mono illness. The drug also shortened the period that the mono bug, Epstein-Barr virus (EBV), could be cultured from the throat washings. Other measures of drug usefulness, such as shortening the duration of fever, were not significantly altered. The possibility that mono will respond to acyclovir capsules is being explored further. We suspect acyclovir will help these patients once the proper dosage and way to give the drug are worked out.

Cytomegalovirus Diseases

Cytomegalovirus is the toughest member of the human herpesvirus family to treat. Efforts to influence favorably the course of CMV infections in infants and transplant patients have uniformly failed during the past 25 years. Medical science learned in the mid-1970s that vidarabine, such a promising drug for herpes simplex infections, did not help kidney transplant patients with CMV disease—it made them even worse. Based on this experience, we were skeptical but desperate in 1980 when we began studying intravenous acyclovir for treatment of CMV infections in transplant patients. We were pleasantly surprised upon completion of the study 18 months later. The patients who had received acyclovir got better faster with significantly fewer days of fever than those who had received the placebo. Because our initial study involved only 16 patients, we are conducting another clinical investigation in which patients receive two weeks of acyclovir rather than one.

The future may be brighter for patients with CMV disease because a derivative of acyclovir has been shown to be 10 times more effective against CMV in laboratory tests. Patients are now receiving this drug in experimental studies. Another drug, arildone, has effectively stopped CMV growth in cell cultures but has not yet been clinically tested against CMV disease.

WHY HAS IT TAKEN SO LONG TO DEVELOP ANTIVIRAL DRUGS?

The development of effective antiviral drugs has lagged 20 to 30 years behind the successful use of antibiotics against bacteria and fungi. Bacteria grow well in artifical nutrients that are easily prepared in the laboratory. But viruses cannot survive outside living cells. Viruses are pirates attacking normal cells, kidnapping their cellular mechanisms and controlling their actions. For many years, scientists could not grow viruses to study except in laboratory animals.

As work toward understanding and preventing polio was intensified in the late 1940s, Dr. John Enders and associates in Boston popularized the use of tissue culture. Tissue culture is a method of growing cells outside the living organism. Once scientists learned to keep cells alive in test tubes, viruses could be easily cultivated. This method of study was simpler and more efficient than use of laboratory animals. Virologists finally were able to observe the effects of the virus on the cell. You can imagine the excitement of those pioneering scientists peering through their microscopes! In a sense, they saw their antagonist for the first time. Recall the saying, "We have met the enemy, and they are ours." Such was the case in virus research.

But the war against viruses still faced a major obstacle because of the viruses' parasitic nature: how do you destroy the virus without destroying the cell in which it lives? If you are successful in eliminating the virions, but damage too many host cells in the process, you may make the patient even sicker than before.

Herpesviruses became a prime target of investigation, not just because their infections are so common, but because their biological structure is complex. In a physical sense, they provide a bigger target to shoot at with biochemical weapons. An approach toward successful therapy was opened when we learned that herpesviruses teach the cell to manufacture special enzymes not found in uninfected cells. Enzymes are dynamic molecules that cause changes in cell activities. Just as generals plan their attack through enemy lines, scientists charted their battle to gain control of the virus. Their strategy: take advantage of the special virus-directed enzymes. This approach could interfere with the viruses' takeover of the normal cell without damaging too many cells in the process. Thus the infection could be cured before the patient suffered serious effects from the viral attack.

HOW DRUGS WORK AGAINST HERPESVIRUSES

DNA, the now familiar acronym for deoxyribonucleic acid, is found in every cell in the human body. It carries vital information on heredity. You might consider DNA as a vault of highly guarded secrets, including the most important secret of all: how to reproduce. Herpesviruses also contain DNA.

Think of DNA as two long rows of alphabet blocks, paired side by side with matching letters, A-A, B-B, C-C, and so forth. Changing any of these blocks would modify the information of the DNA and, ultimately, viral reproduction. Scientists found a way to do this through a clever scientific trick. By placing faulty blocks, mimicking the real ones, in the pile of unused blocks, we can fool the DNA-building enzymes into taking a bogus block. It's like replacing the block marked "A" with a block marked "a." They look similar, but their grammatic function is quite different. When block "a" is added onto the growing chain, the next proper block won't fit in place. The DNA chain can't be finished. Antiviral drugs such as acyclovir, vidarabine, and idoxuridine are all "trick" blocks that break the DNA chain.

Most of you know that our cells constantly manufacture DNA. What is to keep the antiviral tricksters from destroying the DNA of our normal cells? In fact, this happens to a certain extent with many antiherpes drugs. Acyclovir is different because it has no effect on DNA until activated by specific enzymes. In a sense, the drug has to be charged with energy to do the job. The herpes-infected cell is forced to make an enzyme called thymidine kinase, TK for short. TK is a special virus-directed enzyme that scientists have learned to exploit. TK activates acyclovir, making the drug attractive to the enzyme building the viral DNA chain. This DNA-building enzyme then puts the trick acyclovir block on the end of the embryonic viral DNA chain, where it sticks like bubble gum on the sole of your shoe. Acyclovir is bound irreversibly, the chain cannot be finished, and new viral particles are never formed. The TK enzyme becomes a turncoat, deserting its viral ally to become the means of destruction of the virus itself. The battle against the virus is won. Casualties among normal cells are few because acyclovir is never activated within uninfected cells and their DNA is left untouched.

RESISTANCE OF HERPESVIRUSES TO THE ANTIVIRAL DRUGS

Nothing in medicine is more frustrating than suddenly discovering that a drug once 100 percent effective against a microorganism has lost its punch. In the halcyon days of penicillin, when that antibiotic was being used against every infection imaginable, staphylococci quickly learned how to attack and inactivate the molecule. A mad chase ensued for synthesis of penicillinlike compounds that killed the penicillin-resistant staph.

Viruses are simpler than bacteria, but they still can learn to resist drugs designed to destroy them. Shortly after the discovery of acyclovir, scientists found that laboratory strains of herpes simplex could develop resistance to the drug. Doctors worried that acyclovir resistance would spread rapidly among all herpes simplex viruses. Concern was heightened when the case of a seven-year-old boy with weakened immunity was reported in the February 11, 1982, issue of the *New England Journal of Medicine*. Herpes simplex type 1 resistant to acyclovir was isolated from the boy's mouth during a lengthy course of intravenous acyclovir therapy. The research team, headed by Dr. Clyde Crumpacker, commented, "This observation has important implications for the widespread clinical use of acyclovir," and they suggested that intravenous acyclovir might be reserved for "the treatment of very serious or life-threatening infections caused by herpes simplex virus type 1."

The notion of limiting acyclovir, even in the intravenous form, to very severe herpes simplex infections was not warranted on the basis of that single case report. The boy's sores healed in the presence of an apparently resistant virus. When the child died from complications of his damaged immune system, no evidence of herpes was found in his body. Despite its apparent resistance, the virus was eradicated. Several other reports of herpes resistant to acyclovir have been published, but in every case the herpes sores healed—evidence that the resistant viruses do not cause serious herpes disease. I felt so strongly that acyclovir resistance was being exaggerated that I addressed the issue in an editorial for the March 1983 issue of *Annals of Internal Medicine*. Since then,

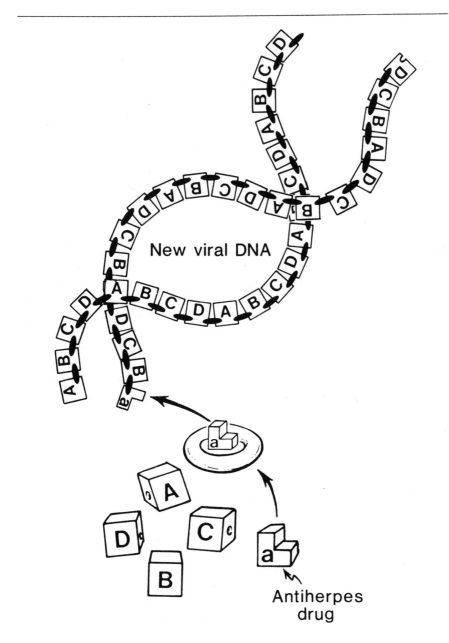

How many antiviral drugs work. As the double-stranded herpesvirus DNA is being formed by matching blocks, an antiviral block "a" is picked up by the doughnut-shaped DNA building enzyme and inserted at the end of the chain. Normal DNA building blocks won't match because of the irregular configuration of the antiherpes drug, and viral DNA cannot be completed.

experience continues to mount supporting my view that "although evidence for development of resistance should be monitored, herpes simplex strains resistant to acyclovir have not been a clinical problem."

"UPPERS" FOR THE IMMUNE SYSTEM

Instead of attacking the virus directly, why not bolster our immune defenses? This approach is reasonable because our battle against herpesviruses is a tug-of-war between our immune systems and the viral invaders.

Interferon

So far interferon has been the most promising of these immune-system "uppers" for viral infections. The exact way that interferon exerts its power is unknown. Herpesviruses cause production of natural interferons immediately after they infect cells. Interferon turns off synthesis of proteins during the early stages of viral replication. It also stimulates special lymphocytes, called natural killer cells, which are vital in host defense against foreign organisms. Finally, interferon seems to prevent the newly formed virus from escaping and invading other cells. Interferon has shown promise against herpes simplex infections of the face, chickenpox, shingles, and cytomegalovirus infections in immuno-suppressed patients. Unlike the antiherpes drugs, interferon can affect more than one virus or one viral family. The development of interferon, however, was severely limited until recently by cost. Now that interferon can be synthesized economically by common bacteria, more will be available for clinical experiments.

Transfer Factor

Transfer factor is another "upper" for the immune system. As the name implies, it transfers the ability to recognize foreign invaders from one white blood cell to another. Exciting work has been reported by Dr. Richard Gehrz of St. Paul Children's Hospital in collaboration with our group at the University of Minnesota. Transfer factor given to infants with congenital CMV restores their immune system's ability to react to CMV, a virus they couldn't recognize without transfer factor.

NONSENSE NOSTRUMS

Because herpesviruses are such pernicious pests, causing symptoms spanning months or even decades, all kinds of remedies have been proposed to whisk them away. These remedies proliferated because no proven treatment was available until recently. Few such herpes potions have been subjected to rigorous clinical trials. Those that have undergone scientific scrutiny all failed their acid test. Some of these quack cures are potentially dangerous. Perhaps the worst of all is the use of repeated smallpox vaccinations. Rather than glorifying any with detailed descriptions, I've made a list of the more popular nostrums that don't work. This list is not all-inclusive; nearly every week a new folk remedy to exorcise herpesviruses comes to our attention.

Drugs, Devices, and Methods INEFFECTIVE in
Herpes of the Lips or Genitals

adenosine monophosphate	levamisole
betadine	neutral red dye
BHT	nonoxynol 9
chloroform	polio vaccine
2-deoxyglucose	proflavine
dimethylsulfoxide (DMSO)	rubella vaccine
electric shock	smallpox (vaccinia) vaccine
ether	tuberculosis (BCG) vaccine
gentian violet	vidarabine cream
influenza vaccine	vitamin B complex
iodine	vitamin C
isoprinosine	vitamin D
L-lysine	

Although the nostrum may appear to cure herpes, our own immune system probably is responsible for the healing. It is sometimes hard to convince people of this fact, however. One patient aired her story in a *Minneapolis Star and Tribune* column on March 14, 1983. She swore that the smallpox vaccination she received more than 20 years earlier temporarily solved her herpes problem. Seeking to balance the report, columnist Jim Klobuchar called me for an opinion. Here's what I told him:

> *There's no evidence that smallpox vaccine for herpes does any good even if it were safe, which of course it isn't. . . . The potentially harmful effects of the vaccine in a small percentage of cases has been known for some time. There have been cases of loss of fingers and toes.*

The columnist conveyed my thoughts to the woman, who responded by saying: "I'm glad to hear his opinion. I disagree. I think smallpox vaccine would cure my cold sores." I agree with Mr. Klobuchar's final comment: "Moses himself had trouble making converts."

A final note on nostrums. In the mid-1950s doctors injected blister fluid from a man's penis into his abdomen as an innovative attempt to treat genital herpes. What do you think happened? The penile sores returned every month, just as before, but, lo and behold, the patient now had recurrent herpes on his belly.

NEWBORNS LIKE JEREMY ADVANCE HERPES RESEARCH

Margaret Miller caught genital herpes in her late teens and experienced relatively mild recurrent episodes until she was 20. She married in 1981 at age 21 and became pregnant within a few months. Margaret informed her obstetrician of her history of genital herpes after reading a frightening magazine story that chronicled a case of neonatal herpes with complications. The obstetrician followed her closely, looking for signs of recurrence, which would necessitate a cesarean section near term to protect the baby from herpes in the vaginal canal. As the time of delivery neared, she attended the doctor's clinic every two weeks for a physical examination and Pap smear. Because the exams and tests remained normal, the doctor decided that Margaret could safely deliver her child vaginally. Margaret went into labor, was admitted to her community hospital, and gave birth to an apparently healthy eight-pound boy who was named Jeremy Jr. after his father.

Jeremy appeared to be developing normally until the third day of life, when an alert pediatrician noted a tiny vesicle on the baby's arm. The physician immediately diagnosed neonatal herpes and placed a frantic call to the University of Minnesota Hospitals in Minneapolis. The University neonatologist and I agreed that the baby should be transferred to our neonatal intensive care unit. Jeremy was rushed to us by ambulance, arriving within three hours of the herpes diagnosis. The child was put in strict isolation because neonatal herpes can spread to other babies in a newborn nursery.

We also noticed that Jeremy had a shrill cry and that his arms and legs were limp, both signs of neurologic infection. To confirm the diagnosis, we removed fluid from the skin lesion. We also swabbed his mouth and eyes and performed a spinal tap. These samples were sent to the virus lab to learn if they contained herpes. But we didn't wait for the results! Because the diagnosis of neonatal herpes was a near certainty, we gave Jeremy experimental antiviral therapy, hoping to kill the virus early enough to prevent permanent damage.

The most difficult task I face as a pediatrician is telling a family that their seemingly healthy newborn child may not grow up to live a long and happy life. In cases of neonatal herpes, the outcome is often tragic. Jeremy's parents were terribly shaken by his diagnosis. At first they were reluctant to believe that he was sick and protested the need for a trip to the University. As I recall, this is a summary of what I told them:

"When no treatment is given, half the babies die of neonatal herpes. Of those who survive, half suffer permanent mental retardation. When the condition is treated, one-quarter of the babies die anyway, but many of the survivors—we don't yet know exactly how many—grow and develop normally.

"Fortunately, medical science has made giant strides in recent years in treating neonatal herpes. We don't have all the answers and we can't save every baby, but more and more children like Jeremy are leaving the hospital as beautiful babies.

"Jeremy is eligible to participate in a randomized study of neonatal herpes treatment. By randomized, I mean he will be assigned by chance to one of two drugs. The drugs are called vidarabine and acyclovir. The drug assignments are in sealed envelopes. Both drugs are given through a needle inserted into a small vein in his scalp. He'll feel a slight discomfort from the needle stick, but this is minor compared with the damage that the herpes virus might do."

The parents signed the necessary consent forms. Drug therapy began within a few hours of Jeremy's admission. More vesicles appeared on his arm and chest the next day, indicating that the virus was still multiplying and spreading. With this development, the parents became anxious, as you can imagine. But I was still hopeful the drug assigned to Jeremy would help and tried to build the family's confidence by praising the mother's openness in telling the doctor about her case of genital herpes. That history had alerted doctors in Jeremy's hometown to look carefully for signs of herpes. I emphasized how important it was to have started treatment early.

One day later, the virus lab called the hospital ward to report that herpes was growing from the skin vesicle *and* from spinal fluid. Jeremy's young brain was being invaded by the invidious herpesviruses.

The baby remained in strict isolation, although no new vesicles erupted after the third day. His lesions soon crusted; his cry and muscle strength became normal. Jeremy showed progressive improvement during the 10 days of treatment. A spinal tap, performed the day before his discharge to check for any evidence of remaining virus, was normal. Apparently the herpes had been treated in time.

Follow-up: Children with neonatal herpes must be followed for several years to be certain that brain damage has not occurred. On return examination one year later, Jeremy was a happy little boy with no signs of recurrent herpes. He spoke several words as he toddled about the examining room. We were delighted to learn that the electro-encephalogram showed normal brain activity.

Comment: Neonatal herpes, one of the most devastating of all herpes infections, is finally showing signs of yielding to antiviral drugs. A national research effort headed by Dr. Richard Whitley is investigating vidarabine and acyclovir treatment. More than 100 cases of neonatal herpes will be needed to *prove* efficacy of one or both drugs. Yet patients like Jeremy convince us that we will conquer herpes diseases in the end.

Jeremy's successful outcome was gratifying, but wouldn't it be better to prevent the disease from happening altogether? The last chapter is devoted to progress in herpes research and outlines the most promising future prospect of all: prevention of herpes diseases with vaccines. I'll discuss some of the perplexing problems in clinical research. For instance, why do we practice deception, disguising the active compound and giving some patients placebos?

Herpes Research:
Progress and Promise

Herpes research is progressing at a feverish pace. The 1980s and 1990s will witness a dramatic proliferation of effective antiviral drugs and vaccines because the basic laboratory tools are available for their development. The first major step has been accomplished: all five human herpesviruses can be grown reliably in the laboratory. We're now manipulating their growth characteristics and genetics, making the viruses work for us instead of against us.

However, an obstacle in the development of antiviral drugs is that almost all viral infections are self-limited. In other words, patients routinely recover from the disease. A drug must be free of nearly every undesirable side effect, or else the patient is better off without it. Genital herpes, for example, is not life-threatening. Therefore, a drug that caused inability to drive a car or memory loss would be unacceptable to most patients with genital herpes. A number of candidate viral drugs have failed to pass muster because of the requirement for minimal toxicity. As a general rule of thumb, the more effective a drug, the more significant its side effects.

Eradication of herpesviruses is especially difficult because all members of the human herpes family establish latency in the host. None of the present antiviral drugs works against latent virus. These drugs fall into two categories: antimetabolites that attack the newly assembling virus, and immune stimulators that enhance our immune attack against the virus. If the virus is not actively multiplying, drugs that inhibit viral metabolism have no target. Likewise, drugs designed to bolster our immune defenses are useless until viruses awaken from their dormant state and provide an enemy for the immune system to engage.

Once a candidate drug has emerged from the array of contenders, studies proceed in stepwise fashion to bring the discovery from the laboratory to the patient. After many years of research, a few compounds have performed well enough in the lab to reach the final step— controlled studies in humans, often involving placebos.

WHY WE USE PLACEBOS IN STUDIES

Placebos are widely used in scientific studies as "controls" to test new drugs. One of the hottest debates in medicine today is appropriate use of the placebo. Both the practicing physician and medical researcher are confronted with hard questions about the ethics of giving patients so-called dummy pills or worthless injections of sugar water. The dialogue has even reached the pages of prominent medical journals as scientists defend use of a placebo to ensure objectivity of their studies. For example, one of our shingles treatment trials was criticized in the November 17, 1983, issue of the *New England Journal of Medicine*:

> To the Editor: *Balfour et al. found acyclovir effective in decreasing the complications of herpes zoster in immunocompromised patients. We are concerned, however, with the ethics of a placebo-controlled trial. . . . Since an available drug, vidarabine, is known to be effective, the use of [a] placebo control may be questioned.*

We replied:

> *Neither vidarabine, nor interferon, nor any other drug was considered standard therapy for zoster during the period of our trial. Therefore, the use of a placebo control was not only ethical but appropriate.*
> *There is always the possibility that the drug under investigation will prove to be worse than no therapy at all. Far from being unethical, the use of a placebo control spares some patients from receiving a potentially toxic compound that may be without therapeutic benefit. For example, if acyclovir had been found to be harmful to patients with zoster (as was the case with cytarabine), it would have been better to have given them placebo.*

Placebos also are used to guarantee the objectivity of medical personnel. In cases where neither the patient nor the medical team can differentiate placebo from the real drug, the study is called double-blind.

THE PLACEBO NEEDS A PERFECT DISGUISE

Why are medical personnel "blinded" in some studies? Doctors, nurses, and other health support staff tend to be unrealistically optimistic. They believe that whatever they do helps the patient. As a result, they may have a certain bias that the test medication works. This can introduce subjectivity into the data-collection forms and skew the results.

Researchers also must be careful not to reveal to their subjects who gets placebo and who gets drug. Here's where blinding or masking techniques come into play. To blind the patient, test drug and placebo must look identical—and taste the same. The story of vitamin C research highlights the need for masking taste as well as color. It also points out the power of suggestion.

In the early 1970s, the National Institutes of Health launched a long-term prospective double-blind study to resolve the controversial issue of the effectiveness of treating the common cold with vitamin C. A total of 311 NIH employees participated. They each received one gram of either ascorbic acid (vitamin C) or lactose placebo in capsules three times a day for nine months. At the onset of a cold, the volunteers were given an additional three grams daily of either a placebo or vitamin C.

When the long-awaited study results were finally published in the March 10, 1975, issue of the *Journal of the American Medical Association*, the researchers offered a surprising conclusion:

> *Analysis of these data showed that ascorbic acid had at best only a minor influence on the duration and severity of colds, and that the effects demonstrated might be explained equally well by a break in the double blind.*

How could *the* definitive study of vitamin C—a possible curative for the most common of all human ailments—be tarnished by a "break" in the protocol?

Early in the study, the NIH researchers learned that some of the volunteers had tasted the contents of their capsules and believed they could differentiate between ascorbic acid and placebo. At the study's conclusion, volunteers were questioned, and it was discovered that they were able to tell what they were receiving. The placebo group experienced a disproportionate dropout rate, presumably because the volunteers realized they were taking an inactive substance and quit the study cold turkey.

In acknowledging the skewed results, the scientists explained:

> *This study was designed during the summer and rushed into operation to take advantage of the rise in upper respiratory infections expected to occur in the fall. There was no time to design, test, and have manufactured a placebo that would be indistinguishable from ascorbic*

acid. It did not occur to the investigators that a substantial number of the volunteers, presumably fully informed about the purpose of the study and the importance of the double blind, would not be able to resist indefinitely the temptation to learn which medication they were taking.

Although the study failed to provide conclusive data on the efficacy of vitamin C, the researchers did give us some valuable insight into the power of suggestion in medical research, and the importance of perfect blinding in trials with endpoints determined by the patient's symptoms:

Did the participants who had less severe and shorter colds than formerly guess correctly that they were receiving ascorbic acid because they expected it to be effective, while those who had more severe colds assumed that they must be taking placebo? Or did those who knew they were taking ascorbic acid or placebo because they had tasted their capsules have less or more severe colds as a result of suggestion?

The scientists were unable to answer their own queries because the number of subjects was too small to draw a definite conclusion. However, ensuing studies with taste-proof capsules failed to show any difference between vitamin C and placebo in treating the common cold.

QUESTIONS ABOUT HERPES RESEARCH
Q. What are the steps in developing a drug against herpes?
A. You begin in the laboratory, using cell cultures to screen many chemicals against herpes. Cell cultures are layers or suspensions of living cells in tubes, plates, or flasks. Virus and experimental drug are added to the cell cultures. You can see if the virus has been killed by examining cells under a light microscope or by holding plates of cells stained with dye to the light and counting plaques (clear areas) that represent live virus. Cell culture experiments provide an initial idea of the drug's therapeutic index: the concentration needed to kill the virus versus that which damages normal cells. If the antiviral dose is similar to the toxic dose in cell cultures, the drug usually is rejected because its side effects likely are too great for clinical safety.

The tissue culture system, although reliable and easier to work with than living animals, is terribly artificial. There are no organs, no blood, no immune system, no natural dynamics. You are simply putting virus and drug together in a liquid medium. If tissue culture results are promising, you progress to animal studies that provide clues about how often to give the drug, how much to give, and what organs may be affected. Unfortunately, drugs work differently in different laboratory animals. In developing a candidate antiviral drug, several animal species are used because a drug may be effective in a guinea pig but not in a dog. Side effects also may be found in one species but not another. Effects of the drug in pregnant animals are checked because some drugs may be safe except during pregnancy. (Recall the thalidamide tragedy several decades ago.) Drugs apparently safe and effective in laboratory studies may then be used in clinical trials.

If the drug has shown significant toxicity, trials may still proceed but involve critically ill patients who have a lot to gain from a therapeutically active drug and therefore are willing to sustain more side effects. For example, a bone marrow transplant patient with CMV pneumonia has at best a 50 percent chance of survival. It would be better to test a candidate CMV drug first in such a patient than in a pregnant woman, who has a very low likelihood of developing CMV and passing the disease on to her baby.

To prove effectiveness, the new compound must be pitted against an existing drug or, if none exists, a placebo. Test results are evaluated impartially using acceptable statistical methods. If the therapeutic benefits outweigh the side effects, the sponsor, usually a pharmaceutical company, may file the data as a new drug application with the FDA. After appropriate evaluation, the FDA may grant the sponsor a license.

Q. Why can't you learn everything you need to know about a new drug from animals?

A. Herpesviruses are found in many animals. Even cats, cattle, and catfish, to name just a few, have their own species of herpesviruses. Herpesviruses cause kidney cancer in frogs and fatal encephalitis in Lippizaner horses. Most animal herpesviruses are of no consequence to people. An exception is herpes simiae, a herpesvirus of monkeys that can produce severe encephalitis in humans. Herpes simiae, also known as herpes B, is a problem only for animal handlers who come in close contact with monkeys.

On the other hand, human herpesviruses do not produce the same diseases in animals that they cause in people. The viruses have become adapted to their specific host through the centuries. Human viruses don't infect and multiply in the natural way in study animals. Therefore, if the virus is killed when mice receive a drug, that does not mean the drug works in people.

Q. Why don't you use other primates? Isn't the biological makeup of the chimpanzee almost identical to that of the human being?

A. *Almost* identical does not mean identical. For example, monkeys suffer from their own kind of smallpox, but it's a very mild infection and they recover uneventfully. We are trying to develop a chickenpox vaccine in people, but we can't learn much from monkeys because they don't get sick from chickenpox. Nevertheless, in some respects monkeys are better research subjects than rodents. Monkey experiments were instrumental in finding a cure for polio, because monkeys, like people, develop paralysis from poliovirus.

Q. **Is it fair to exclude someone from a study that might help them if they don't meet your enrollment requirements to a T? For instance, what if I've had herpes for four days, and you're looking for patients who have had it for three?**

A. You cannot make exceptions after the study protocol has been established, or else the study invalidates itself. The crucial phase of any clinical experiment is the time when the patient begins to show improvement. Critical changes generally occur in the first three or four days of a disease. Therefore, if you accept late-entering patients, you do not have enough time to show changes. You must select a group of patients in whom changes can be demonstrated. We conduct a clinical trial because we don't know for sure that the drug works. Theoretically, the risk of a drug could be greater than no drug at all, as I mentioned in the section "Why We Use Placebos in Studies."

Q. **How many patients do you need to make a study significant?**

A. It all depends on what you're looking for. Biomedical statisticians are called on to decide the "sample size." Both statistical significance and clinical significance matter. If you're looking for one day less pain, you probably won't need as many patients as in a study looking for three days less pain. The key question: is one day less pain of sufficient benefit to the average patient? Probably not.

When undertaking a study, there are also some practical matters to consider, such as the amount of funds available for clinical care and the time staff can devote to the project. The more patients studied, the greater the cost and time commitment, but the less the likelihood of claiming an effect that happened by chance.

Q. **Do you ever stop a study before its planned conclusion?**

A. Yes. If you run into apparent problems with drug toxicity or if every patient enrolled gets sicker, you must curtail the research and learn as quickly as possible if the ill effects were due to the new drug, the disease itself, or other complications.

Q. **Should patients be paid to particpate in a study?**

A. Sometimes, yes. I believe it is appropriate to pay patients for their inconvenience. But if the financial reward is too great, you may be coercing people and that is unethical. Is the inducement so large that the patients are unable to judge their own welfare? If so, patients cannot give logical informed consent. In one of our shingles studies, adult patients received $100—a modest amount, I believe, in view of the fact that they came to the hospital emergency room three times a day for a week to undergo a total of 15 intravenous injections. Offering children an honorarium of $100 might be too great a reward, because that seems like a fortune to a child.

HERPES VACCINE—NEW HOPE, NEW CHALLENGE

Early treatment of herpesvirus diseases with antiviral drugs may limit or eliminate virions destined to escape their initial encounter with host defenses. But recognizing each and every first herpes infection soon enough to prevent establishment of latency is impossible. Vaccines hold more promise for eliminating herpesvirus diseases entirely.

Viral vaccines contain antigens—whole or partial virions—that stimulate an immune response in the recipient. Experimental vaccines have been developed against all five members of the human herpesvirus family. As discussed in chapter 5, Japanese investigators have produced a live, attenuated chickenpox vaccine. Chickenpox vaccine trials are proceeding slowly in the United States. Vaccine first was tested exclusively in leukemic children for whom chickenpox is life threatening. The leukemic children did mount an immune response to the vaccine. Vaccine currently is being given experimentally to normal children in the hope that it will prevent chickenpox without producing undesirable side effects or an increased incidence of shingles.

Why is chickenpox vaccine ahead of the other herpesvirus vaccines? A live herpesvirus vaccine has the potential to multiply in the patient, establish latency, and later promote the growth of cancer. Varicella-zoster virus has the most tenuous link to cancer of all the herpes group viruses. The cancer risk from a live chickenpox vaccine is theoretically much less than that from a live herpes simplex vaccine. Therefore, researchers are more comfortable giving chickenpox vaccine to children.

Cytomegalovirus (CMV) vaccine trials (discussed in chapter 8) have been limited mainly to kidney transplant candidates who have major problems with CMV after transplantation. Healthy adults, such as nurses in pediatric intensive care units who come in contact with congenitally infected babies, also have received CMV vaccine experimentally. The

CMV vaccine now being tested is live. Perhaps the CMV vaccine of the future will be made up of only a part of the virus, thus evading the major concern in the development of herpesvirus vaccines—cancer from the vaccine itself.

Because of the presumed association of herpes simplex with human genital cancers, I do not believe that a live herpes vaccine will ever reach clinical trial. Our hope for a successful herpes vaccine rests with killed or subunit vaccines. These vaccines do not reproduce, cannot establish latency, and therefore are inherently safer than live vaccines.

Unfortunately, vaccines made from whole virus particles killed by exposure to formalin or ultraviolet light have been only moderately effective. Killed vaccines are always given unnaturally, that is, beneath the skin or into a muscle. Herpes usually enters through the mouth or genital tract. Therefore, our body's immune system does not encounter the killed virus in the normal way. Local immune defenses in the mouth or genital tract never "see" and learn to recognize the virus. After immunization, killed viral particles remain at the site of inoculation because they cannot multiply to produce a generalized infection. The magnitude of the viral attack is minimal, and the host immune response modest. The immune system's memory cells are weakly imprinted. Immunity provided by most killed viral vaccines wanes after several years.

Subunit vaccines, made from part of the whole virus, are more promising than killed vaccines. Various viral subunits can be tested in laboratory animals, and the component that best stimulates the immune system chosen as the candidate vaccine. The outside coat of herpes simplex which contains glycoproteins (molecules of sugar and protein), is a strong antigen that readily stimulates the immune system. Subunit glycoprotein vaccines for herpes type 1 and type 2 have been produced by scientists at Merck, Sharp & Dohme Research Laboratories in Pennsylvania. The herpes type 2 vaccine induced immune responses in laboratory animals and in some volunteers. More extensive clinical trials are now under way. Data on protection of human subjects against herpes simplex infections and side effects of the vaccine are not yet available.

Candidate herpes vaccines have been produced by recombinant DNA (gene-splicing) technology. Scientists at Molecular Genetics Inc., Minnetonka, Minnesota, discovered a herpes simplex gene responsible for the production of an important part of the viral coat. This gene was spliced into whole bacteria. As the bacteria reproduce in broth cultures, they manufacture the herpes gene product along with themselves. That herpes-specific protein antigen made within the bacteria is then purified and used as a vaccine. This method is less expensive than growing viruses in tissue cultures and purifying whole virions. The bacteria-produced vaccine is "cleaner" because there is absolutely no chance of contamination by live viruses that might survive after the preparation of a killed whole virus vaccine.

Another approach to herpes vaccine production involves the marriage of classic immunization practice with modern DNA technology. The word *vaccine* is derived from *vaccinia*, the name of the cowpox virus strain first used by Dr. Edward Jenner 200 years ago to immunize against smallpox. Vaccination against smallpox continued until worldwide eradication of the disease was accomplished in the mid-1970s. Researchers at the New York State Department of Health have inserted genes from herpes simplex and hepatitis B viruses into vaccinia. They plan to use the live vaccinia vaccine to produce the proteins that will stimulate immunity against hepatitis B and herpes.

This novel approach may not be completely safe. Physicians involved in routine immunization of children recall that smallpox vaccination was associated with significant side effects. Some children developed a generalized infection resembling chickenpox. Others scratched their primary vaccination site and spread the virus all over their bodies, resulting in multiple pocklike scars. The vaccinia vehicle for the herpes gene theoretically could produce a rash worse than herpes itself.

Recombinant DNA techniques offer new hope for inexpensive, effective herpes vaccines. Vaccines hold the greatest promise for preventing first episodes of herpes infections, and thus their value could increase with each successive generation of use. The challenge: vaccines might prevent primary herpes diseases, but their ability to suppress recurrences is questionable. If our natural immune defenses can't ward off recurrences, why should artifical stimulation be effective? Vaccines might be worthless for the estimated nine million Americans already suffering from recurrent genital herpes. Experience with live CMV vaccine indicates that primary CMV disease can be modified but that patients infected before immunization experience reactivation of their own CMV after transplantation.

The timetable for development and licensure of a genital herpes vaccine is blurred by uncertainties, the most important being the therapeutic index of the vaccine—the ratio of its effectiveness versus

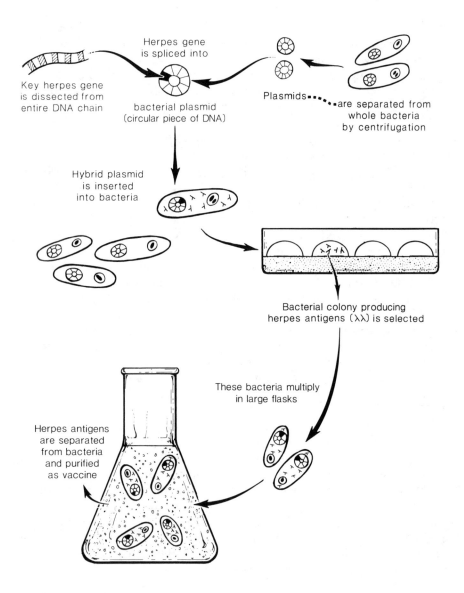

Herpes gene
is spliced into

Key herpes gene
is dissected from
entire DNA chain

bacterial plasmid
(circular piece of DNA)

Plasmids••••••are separated from
whole bacteria
by centrifugation

Hybrid plasmid
is inserted
into bacteria

Bacterial colony producing
herpes antigens (λλ) is selected

These bacteria multiply
in large flasks

Herpes antigens
are separated
from bacteria
and purified
as vaccine

Gene-splicing (recombinant DNA) method utilizing common bacteria to produce herpes vaccine.

side effects. My best guess is that if any of the candidate herpes vaccines are shown to be protective and safe they will not be available to the general public until about 1990.

Is Herpes Vaccine for You?

Many of you may want to participate in vaccine tests. Proper studies will be rigorously conducted and most likely will be double-blind and placebo-controlled. Are these studies appropriate for you? Clinical trials are not for everyone. A substantial amount of time is required, especially at the beginning of the study. Many potential subjects find their occupations too demanding for them to become involved in a clinical investigation.

An integral part of the agreement between patient and physician-investigator is that once enrolled, the patient makes every effort to complete the study. Patients whose attitude is "I'll give this a try for a day or two and see if I like it" should not participate.

The investigators, on the other hand, have an obligation to explain clearly the design and conduct of the study, and what they hope to learn. If you don't understand any part of the protocol, don't be afraid to ask any question on your mind *before you participate*. The most satisfactory relationship between volunteer and investigator results from a thorough understanding of each other's role in the project.

I believe the most important attribute for a subject in a clinical trial is intellectual curiosity about medical science. Most of our study patients want to advance medical knowledge. Although naturally concerned about their own illness, they realize that what is being evaluated may not work for them. Ask yourself this question before you volunteer for a study: if the test drug is ultimately proved ineffective against my disease, would I still be willing to take it? In other words, would you consider your participation an important research contribution regardless of any personal gain that you might derive? If your answer is yes, you are an ideal person for a clinical trial. And clinical testing is the culmination of applied science, the final giant step that brings virology research from the bench to the bedside.

Epilogue / 169

Herpes diseases are among the commonest of human infections. Through evolution, herpesviruses have learned to survive—indeed flourish—intimately with their human hosts. Coexisting with herpesviruses is not always easy, because latent virions inside our cells retain their potential to reactivate, resulting in recurrent disease. As we age, herpesviruses are like rites of passage, causing cold sores and chickenpox in children, mononucleosis in adolescents, genital herpes in young adults, and shingles in the elderly.

How can we cope with the herpes diseases that affect our health? First, forget the myths. You can't get herpes from a handshake, public toilet seats are safe; and women with genital herpes can deliver perfectly healthy babies. Herpesviruses are caught through intimate contact. Their spread can be stopped by following the practical guidelines in this book. And the prospect of acquiring permanent protection through immunization is becoming a reality—vaccines against chickenpox, cytomegalovirus, and herpes are being tested now in volunteers.

If you're already infected, remember: **herpes diseases are self-limited and manageable.** The majority of herpes diseases can be treated, and treated again if they recur. The difference between treatment and cure is semantic so long as the treatment remains effective—which in the case of genital herpes it does. All five human herpesviruses are vulnerable to selective attack. New therapies are providing our immune systems with an increasingly greater advantage in the battle against these viral invaders. Even immunosuppressed cancer and transplant patients can conquer herpes diseases with the aid of antiviral drugs.

A few herpes diseases—such as postherpetic neuralgia—have eluded specific therapy. But researchers are determined to find effective treatments with the help of dedicated patients who willingly participate in clinical studies. Antiviral drugs now being tested against acute shingles show real promise for lessening the pain of postherpetic neuralgia. It is conceivable that chickenpox vaccine could prevent shingles from ever happening.

Research on prevention and treatment of herpes diseases is progressing swiftly. Rapid advances have been made possible only because men, women, and children donated their time, their trust, and even their bodies to medical science. I'm speaking of the volunteer patients who are the heroes of this book. They are the Monicas, the Teds, and babies like Jeremy. They give unselfishly of themselves so that some day we may be entirely free from the herpes family legacy of physical and social misery.

Selected References

Selected References / 173

The following references, subdivided by subject, were selected from approximately 300 used to compile this book. These articles and symposia were chosen because they contain original observations published in the professional medical literature. Medical libraries will permit you to read the references and will provide photocopies at a nominal charge. Public libraries carry some medical books and journals, and your librarian may be able to obtain others on request.

ANTIVIRAL THERAPY

Arvin, A. M., J. H. Kushner, S. Feldman, R. L. Baehner, D. Hammond, and T. C. Merigan. "Human Leukocyte Interferon for the Treatment of Varicella in Children with Cancer." *New England Journal of Medicine* 306 (1982):761–65.

Balfour, H. H., Jr. "Intravenous Acyclovir Therapy for Varicella in Immunocompromised Children." *Journal of Pediatrics* 104 (1984):134–36.

Balfour, H. H., Jr. "Resistance of Herpes Simplex to Acyclovir." *Annals of Internal Medicine* 98 (1983):404–6. [Editorial]

Balfour, H. H., Jr., B. Bean, O. L. Laskin, R. F. Ambinder, J. D. Meyers, J. C. Wade, J. A. Zaia, D. Aeppli, L. E. Kirk, A. C. Segreti, R. E. Keeney, and the Burroughs Wellcome Collaborative Acyclovir Study Group. "Acyclovir Halts Progression of Herpes Zoster in Immunocompromised Patients." *New England Journal of Medicine* 308 (1983):1448–53.

Bean B., C. Braun, and H. H. Balfour, Jr. "Acyclovir Therapy for Acute Herpes Zoster." *Lancet* 2 (1982):118–21.

Bierman, S. M., W. Kirkpatrick, and H. Fernandez. "Clinical Efficacy of Ribavirin in the Treatment of Genital Herpes Simplex Virus Infection." *Chemotherapy* 27 (1981):139–45.

Bryson, Y. J., M. Dillon, M. Lovett, G. Acuna, S. Taylor, J. D. Cherry, B. L. Johnson, E. Wiesmeier, W. Growdon, T. Creagh-Kirk, and R. Keeney. "Treatment of First Episodes of Genital Herpes Simplex Virus Infection with Oral Acyclovir: A Randomized Double-Blind Controlled Trial in Normal Subjects." *New England Journal of Medicine* 308 (1983):916–21.

Corey, L., K. H. Fife, J. K. Benedetti, C. A. Winter, A. Fahnlander, J. D. Connor, M. A. Hintz, and K. K. Holmes. "Intravenous Acyclovir for the Treatment of Primary Genital Herpes." *Annals of Internal Medicine* 98 (1983):914–21.

Corey, L., A. J. Nahmias, M. E. Guinan, J. K. Benedetti, C. W. Critchlow, and K. K. Holmes. "A Trial of Topical Acyclovir in Genital Herpes Simplex Virus Infections." *New England Journal of Medicine* 306 (1982):1313–19.

Crumpacker, C. S., L. E. Schnipper, S. I. Marlowe, P. N. Kowalsky, B. J. Hershey, and M. J. Levin. "Resistance to Antiviral Drugs of Herpes Simplex Virus Isolated from a Patient Treated with Acyclovir." *New England Journal of Medicine* 306 (1982):343–46.

Elion, G. B., P. A. Furman, J. A. Fyfe, P. de Miranda, L. Beauchamp, and H. J. Schaeffer. "Selectivity of Action of an Antiherpetic Agent, 9-(2-hydroxyethoxymethyl)guanine." *Proceedings of the National Academy of Sciences, USA* 74 (1977):5716–20.

Fiddian, A. P., and L. Ivanyi. "Topical Acyclovir in the Management of Recurrent Herpes Labialis." *British Journal of Dermatology* 109 (1983):321–26.

Fiddian, A. P., J. M. Yeo, R. Stubbings, and D. Dean. "Successful Treatment of Herpes Labialis with Topical Acyclovir." *British Medical Journal* 286 (1983):1699–1701.

Field, H. J., and I. Phillips, editors. "Acyclovir." *Journal of Antimicrobial Chemotherapy* 12 (Suppl B) (1983).

Hanto, D. W., G. Frizzera, K. J. Gajl-Peczalska, K. Sakamoto, D. T. Purtilo, H. H. Balfour, Jr., R. L. Simmons, and J. S. Najarian. "Epstein-Barr Virus-Induced B-cell Lymphoma after Renal Transplantation: Acyclovir Therapy and Transition from Polyclonal to Monoclonal B-cell Proliferation." *New England Journal of Medicine* 306 (1982):913–18.

Hirsch, M. S., and R. T. Schooley. "Treatment of Herpesvirus Infections." *New England Journal of Medicine* 309 (1983):963–70 and 1034–39.

Hirsch M. S., R. T. Schooley, A. B. Cosimi, P. S. Russell, F. L. Delmonico, N. E. Tolkoff-Rubin, J. T. Herrin, K. Cantell, M.-L. Farrell, T. R. Rota, and R. H. Rubin. "Effects of Interferon-Alpha on Cytomegalovirus Reactivation Syndromes in Renal-Transplant Recipients." *New England Journal of Medicine* 308 (1983):1489–93.

Jeffries, D. J., and A. S. Tyms. "Arildone, a Potent Inhibitor of Cytomegalovirus Replication." *Lancet* 1 (1983):1214–15. [Letter]

Karlowski, T. R., T. C. Chalmers, L. D. Frenkel, A. Z. Kapikian, T. L. Lewis, and J. M. Lynch. "Ascorbic Acid for the Common Cold: A Prophylactic and Therapeutic Trial." *Journal of the American Medical Association* 231 (1975):1038–42.

King, D. H., and G. Galasso, editors. *Proceedings of a Symposium on Acyclovir. American Journal of Medicine* 73(A) (1982).

Marker, S. C., R. J. Howard, K. E. Groth, A. R. Mastri, R. L. Simmons, J. S. Najarian, and H. H. Balfour, Jr. "A Trial of Vidarabine for Cytomegalovirus Infection in Renal Transplant Patients." *Archives of Internal Medicine* 140 (1980):1441–44.

Merigan, T. C., K. H. Rand, R. B. Pollard, P. S. Abdallah, G. W. Jordan, and R. P. Fried. "Human Leukocyte Interferon for the Treatment of Herpes Zoster in Patients with Cancer." *New England Journal of Medicine* 298 (1978):981–87.

Mindel, A., M. W. Adler, S. Sutherland, and A. P. Fiddian. "Intravenous Acyclovir Treatment for Primary Genital Herpes." *Lancet* 1 (1982):697–700.

Mitchell, C. D., B. Bean, S. R. Gentry, K. E. Groth, J. R. Boen, and H. H. Balfour, Jr. "Acyclovir Therapy for Mucocutaneous Herpes Simplex Infections in Immunocompromised Patients." *Lancet* 1 (1981):1389–92.

Nilsen, A. E., T. Aasen, A. M. Halsos, B. R. Kinge, E. A. L. Tjotta, K. Wikstrom, and A. P. Fiddian. "Efficacy of Oral Acyclovir in the Treatment of Initial and Recurrent Genital Herpes." *Lancet* 2 (1982):571–73.

Pavan-Langston, D., R. A. Buchanan, and C. A. Alford, Jr., editors. *Adenine Arabinoside: An Antiviral Agent.* New York: Raven Press, 1975.

Pazin, G. J., J. A. Armstrong, M. T. Lam, G. C. Tarr, P. J. Jannetta, and M. Ho. "Prevention of Reactivated Herpes Simplex Infection by Human Leukocyte Interferon After Operation on the Trigeminal Root." *New England Journal of Medicine* 301 (1979):225–30.

Reichman, R. C., G. J. Badger, G. J. Mertz, L. Corey, D. D. Richman, J. D. Connor, D. Redfield, M. C. Savoia, M. N. Oxman, Y. Bryson, D. L. Tyrrell, J. Portnoy, T. Creigh-Kirk, R. E. Keeney, T. Ashikaga, and R. Dolin. "Treatment of Recurrent Genital Herpes

Simplex Infections with Oral Acyclovir: A Controlled Trial." *Journal of the American Medical Association* 251 (1984):2103–2107.

Spruance, S. L., L. E. Schnipper, J. C. Overall, Jr., E. R. Kern, B. Wester, J. Modlin, G. Wenerstrom, C. Burton, K. A. Arndt, G. L. Chiu, and C. S. Crumpacker. "Treatment of Herpes Simplex Labialis with Topical Acyclovir in Polyethylene Glycol." *Journal of Infectious Diseases* 146 (1982):85–90.

Stevens, D. A., G. W. Jordan, T. F. Waddell, and T. C. Merigan. "Adverse Effect of Cytosine Arabinoside on Disseminated Zoster in a Controlled Trial." *New England Journal of Medicine* 289 (1973):873–78.

Whitley, R. J., L. T. Ch'ien, R. Dolin, G. J. Galasso, C. A. Alford, Jr., and the NIAID Collaborative Antiviral Study Group. "Adenine Arabinoside Therapy of Herpes Zoster in the Immunosuppressed." *New England Journal of Medicine* 294 (1976):1193–99.

Whitley, R. J., M. Hilty, R. Haynes, Y. Bryson, J. D. Connor, S.-J. Soong, C. A. Alford, Jr., and the [NIAID] Collaborative [Antiviral] Study Group. "Vidarabine Therapy of Varicella in Immunosuppressed Patients." *Journal of Pediatrics* 101 (1982): 125–31.

Whitley, R. J., S.-J. Soong, R. Dolin, R. Betts, C. Linnemann, Jr., C. A. Alford, Jr., and [NIAID] the Collaborative [Antiviral] Study Group. "Early Vidarabine Therapy to Control the Complications of Herpes Zoster in Immunosuppressed Patients." *New England Journal of Medicine* 307 (1982):971–75.

Whitley, R. J., S.-J. Soong, R. Dolin, G. J. Galasso, L. T. Ch'ien, C. A. Alford, Jr., and the NIAID Collaborative Antiviral Study Group. "Adenine Arabinoside Therapy of Biopsy-Proved Herpes Simplex Encephalitis." *New England Journal of Medicine* 297 (1977):289–94.

CANCER

Kaufman R. H., G. R. Dreesman, J. Burek, M. O. Korhonen, D. O. Matson, J. L. Melnick, K. L. Powell, D. J. M. Purifoy, R. J. Courtney, and E. Adam. "Herpesvirus-Induced Antigens in Squamous-Cell Carcinoma in Situ of the Vulva." *New England Journal of Medicine* 305 (1981):483–88.

Kessler, I. I. "Etiological Concepts in Cervical Carcinogenesis." *Gynecologic Oncology* 12 (1981):S7–S24.

Martin, C. E. "Marital and Coital Factors in Cervical Cancer." *American Journal of Public Health* 57 (1967):803–14.

Rapp, F., and R. Duff. "Oncogenic Conversion of Normal Cells by Inactivated Herpes Simplex Viruses." *Cancer* 34 (1974):1353–62.

zur Hausen H. "Human Genital Cancer: Synergism between Two Virus Infections or Synergism between a Virus Infection and Initiating Events?" *Lancet* 2 (1982):1370–72.

CHICKENPOX AND SHINGLES

Balfour, H. H., Jr., K. E. Groth, J. McCullough, J. M. Kalis, S. C. Marker, M. E. Nesbit, R. L. Simmons, and J. S. Najarian. "Prevention or Modification of Varicella Using Zoster Immune Plasma." *American Journal of Diseases of Children*. 131 (1977):693–96.

Groth, K. E., J. McCullough, and H. H. Balfour, Jr. "Varicella Immunity in Adults." *Minnesota Medicine* 63 (1980):87–89.

Leclair, J. M., J. A. Zaia, M. J. Levin, R. G. Congdon, and D. A. Goldmann. "Airborne Transmission of Chickenpox in a Hospital." *New England Journal of Medicine* 302 (1980):450–53.

Pancoast, H. K., and E. P. Pendergrass. "The Occurrence of Herpes Zoster in Hodgkin's Disease." *American Journal of The Medical Sciences* 168 (1924):326–34.

Ragozzino, M. W., L. J. Melton, III, L. T. Kurland, C. P. Chu, and H. O. Perry. "Population-Based Study of Herpes Zoster and Its Sequelae." *Medicine* 61 (1982):310–16.

Reye, R. D. K., G. Morgan, and J. Baral. "Encephalopathy and Fatty Degeneration of the Viscera: A Disease Entity in Childhood." *Lancet* 2 (1963):749–52.

Weller, T. H. "Varicella and Herpes Zoster: Changing Concepts of the Natural History, Control, and Importance of a Not-So-Benign Virus." *New England Journal of Medicine* 309 (1983):1362–67 and 1434–40.

CYTOMEGALOVIRUS INFECTIONS

Dworsky, M. E., K. Welch, G. Cassady, and S. Stagno. "Occupational Risk for Primary Cytomegalovirus Infection among Pediatric Health-Care Workers." *New England Journal of Medicine* 309 (1983):950–53.

Farber, S., and S. B. Wolbach. "Intranuclear and Cytoplasmic Inclusions (Protozoan-Like Bodies) in the Salivary Glands and Other Organs of Infants." *American Journal of Pathology* 8 (1932):123–35.

Gehrz, R. C., S. C. Marker, S. O. Knorr, J. M. Kalis, and H. H. Balfour, Jr. "Specific Cell-Mediated Immune Defect in Active Cytomegalovirus Infection of Young Children and Their Mothers." *Lancet* 2 (1977):844–47.

Gravell, M., W. T. London, S. A. Houff, D. L. Madden, M. C. Dalakas, J. L. Sever, K. G. Osborn, D. H. Maul, R. V. Henrickson, P. A. Marx, N. W. Lerche, S. Prahalada, and M. B. Gardner. "Transmission of Simian Acquired Immunodeficiency Syndrome (SAIDS) with Blood or Filtered Plasma." *Science* 223 (1984):74–76.

Huang, E.-S., C. A. Alford, Jr., D. W. Reynolds, S. Stagno, and R. F. Pass. "Molecular Epidemiology of Cytomegalovirus Infections in Women and Their Infants." *New England Journal of Medicine* 303 (1980):958–62.

Peckham, C. S., K. S. Chin, J. C. Coleman, K. Henderson, R. Hurley, P. M. Preece. "Cytomegalovirus Infection in Pregnancy: Preliminary Findings from a Prospective Study." *Lancet* 1 (1983):1352–55.

Plotkin, S. A., S. Michelson, and J. Pagano, editors. *CMV: Pathogenesis and Prevention of Human Infection.* New York: Alan R. Liss, 1984.

Simmons, R. L., C. Lopez, H. H. Balfour, Jr., J. M. Kalis, L. C. Rattazzi, and J. S. Najarian. "Cytomegalovirus: Clinical Virological Correlations in Renal Transplant Recipients." *Annals of Surgery* 180 (1974):623–34.

Stagno, S., R. F. Pass, M. E. Dworsky, and C. A. Alford, Jr. "Maternal Cytomegalovirus Infection and Perinatal Transmission." *Clinical Obstetrics and Gynecology* 25 (1982): 563–76.

Stagno, S., R. F. Pass, M. E. Dworsky, R. E. Henderson, E. G. Moore, P. D. Walton, and C. A. Alford, Jr. "Congenital Cytomegalovirus Infection: The Relative Importance of Primary and Recurrent Maternal Infection." *New England Journal of Medicine* 306 (1982):945–49.

Stagno, S., D. W. Reynolds, E.-S. Huang, S. D. Thames, R. J. Smith, and C. A. Alford, Jr. "Congenital Cytomegalovirus Infection: Occurrence in an Immune Population." *New England Journal of Medicine* 296 (1977):1254–58.

HERPES SIMPLEX INFECTIONS

Balfour H. H., Jr., and L. A. Lockman. "Herpesvirus Hominis Type 1 Encephalitis Following Herpes Keratitis." *American Journal of Diseases of Children* 126 (1973):357–59

Balfour, H. H., Jr., M. K. Loken, and M. E. Blaw. "Brain Scan in a Patient with Herpes Simplex Encephalitis." *Journal of Pediatrics* 71 (1967):404–7.

Bugge, I. "The Emotional Impact of Herpes." A Boynton Health Service publication, University of Minnesota, October 1983.

Centers for Disease Control. "Genital Herpes Infection–United States, 1966–1979." *Morbidity and Mortality Weekly Report* 31 (1982):137–39.

Chuang, T.-Y., W. P. D. Su, H. O. Perry, D. M. Ilstrup, and L. T. Kurland. "Incidence and Trend of Herpes Progenitalis: A 15-Year Population Study." *Mayo Clinic Proceedings* 58 (1983):436–41.

Corey, L., H. G. Adams, Z. A. Brown, and K. K. Holmes. "Genital Herpes Simplex Virus Infections: Clinical Manifestations, Course, and Complications." *Annals of Internal Medicine* 98 (1983):958–72.

Corey, L., and K. K. Holmes. "Genital Herpes Simplex Virus Infections: Current Concepts in Diagnosis, Therapy, and Prevention." *Annals of Internal Medicine* 98 (1983):973–83.

Douglas, J. M., and L. Corey. "Fomites and Herpes Simplex Viruses: A Case for Non-venereal Transmission?" *Journal of the American Medical Association* 250 (1983):3093–94. [Editorial]

Goodell, S. E., T. C. Quinn, E. Mkrtichian, M. D. Schuffler, K. K. Holmes, and L. Corey. "Herpes Simplex Virus Proctitis in Homosexual Men: Clinical, Sigmoidoscopic, and Histopathological Features." *New England Journal of Medicine* 308 (1983):868–71.

Greaves, W. L., A. B. Kaiser, R. H. Alford, and W. Schaffner. "The Problem of Herpetic Whitlow among Hospital Personnel." *Infection Control* 1 (1980):381–85.

Hendricks, A. A., and E. P. Shapiro. "Primary Herpes Simplex Infection Following Mouth-to-Mouth Resuscitation." *Journal of the American Medical Association* 243 (1980):257–58.

Knox, S. R., L. Corey, H. A. Blough, and A. M. Lerner. "Historical Findings in Subjects from a High Socioeconomic Group Who Have Genital Infections with Herpes Simplex Virus." *Sexually Transmitted Diseases* 9 (1982):15–20.

Knox, S. R., B. Mandel, and R. Lazarowicz. "Profile of Callers to the VD National Hotline." *Sexually Transmitted Diseases* 8 (1981):245–54.

Larson, T., and Y. Bryson. "Fomites and Herpes Simplex Virus: The Toilet Seat Revisited." *Pediatric Research* 16 (1982):244A. [Abstract]

Linnemann, C. C., Jr., T. G. Buchman, I. J. Light, J. L. Ballard, and B. Roizman. "Transmission of Herpes-Simplex Virus Type 1 in a Nursery for the Newborn: Identification of Viral Isolates by D.N.A. 'Fingerprinting'." *Lancet* 1 (1978):964–66.

Nahmias, A. J., and W. R. Dowdle. "Antigenic and Biologic Differences in Herpesvirus Hominis." *Progress in Medical Virology* 10 (1968):110–59.

Nerurkar, L. S., F. West, M. Day, D. L. Madden, and J. L. Sever. "Survival of Herpes Simplex Virus in Water Specimens Collected from Hot Tubs in Spa Facilities and on Plastic Surfaces." *Journal of the American Medical Association* 250 (1983):3081–83.

Pazin, G. J., M. Ho, and P. J. Jannetta. "Reactivation of Herpes Simplex Virus after Decompression of the Trigeminal Nerve Root." *Journal of Infectious Diseases* 138 (1978):405–9.

Spruance, S. L., J. C. Overall, Jr., E. R. Kern, G. G. Krueger, V. Pliam, and W. Miller. "The Natural History of Recurrent Herpes Simplex Labialis: Implications for Antiviral Therapy." *New England Journal of Medicine* 297 (1977):69–75.

Sullivan-Bolyai, J., H. F. Hull, C. Wilson, and L. Corey. "Neonatal Herpes Simplex Virus Infection in King County, Washington: Increasing Incidence and Epidemiologic Correlates." *Journal of the American Medical Association* 250 (1983):3059–62.

Whitley R. J., A. J. Nahmias, A. M. Visintine, C. L. Fleming, and C. A. Alford, Jr. "The Natural History of Herpes Simplex Virus Infection of Mother and Newborn." *Pediatrics* 66 (1980):489–94.

Whitley, R. J., S.-J. Soong, C. Linneman, Jr., C. Liu, G. Pazin, C. A. Alford, Jr., and the NIAID Collaborative Antiviral Study Group. "Herpes Simplex Encephalitis: Clinical Assessment." *Journal of the American Medical Association* 247 (1982):317–20.

MONO AND OTHER DISEASES CAUSED BY EPSTEIN-BARR VIRUS

Hallee, T. J., A. S. Evans, J. C. Niederman, C. M. Brooks, and J. H. Voegtly. "Infectious Mononucleosis at the United States Military Academy: A Prospective Study of a Single Class over Four Years." *Yale Journal of Biology and Medicine* 3 (1974):182–95.

Hanto, D. W., G. Frizzera, K. Gajl-Peczalska, D. T. Purtilo, G. Klein, R. L. Simmons, and J. S. Najarian. "The Epstein-Barr virus (EBV) in the pathogenesis of posttransplant lymphoma." *Transplant Proceedings* 13 (1981):756–60.

Hanto, D. W., K. Sakamoto, D. T. Purtilo, R. L. Simmons, and J. S. Najarian. "The Epstein-Barr Virus in the Pathogenesis of Posttransplant Lymphoproliferative Disorders." *Surgery* 90 (1981):204–13.

Henle, G., W. Henle, and V. Diehl. "Relation of Burkitt's Tumor-Associated Herpes-Type Virus to Infectious Mononucleosis." *Proceedings of the National Academy of Sciences, USA* 59 (1968):94–101.

Horwitz, C. A., W. Henle, G. Henle, H. Polesky, H. H. Balfour, Jr., R. A. Siem, S. Borken, and P. C. J. Ward. "Heterophil-Negative Infectious Mononucleosis and Mononucleosis-like Illnesses: Laboratory Confirmation of 43 cases." *American Journal of Medicine* 63 (1977):947–57.

Sprunt, T. P., and F. A. Evans. "Mononuclear Leucocytosis in Reaction to Acute Infections ('Infectious Mononucleosis')." *Johns Hopkins Hospital Bulletin* 31 (1920):410–16.

University Health Physicians and P.H.L.S. Laboratories. "Infectious Mononucleosis and Its Relationship to EB Virus Antibody." *British Medical Journal* 2 (1971):643–46.

VACCINES

Asano, Y., P. Albrecht, L. K. Vujcic, G. V. Quinnan, Jr., K. Kawakami, and M. Takahashi. "Five-Year Follow-Up Study of Recipients of Live Varicella Vaccine Using Enhanced Neutralization and Fluorescent Antibody Membrane Antigen Assays." *Pediatrics* 72 (1983):291–94.

Hilleman, M. R., V. M. Larson, E. D. Lehman, R. A. Salerno, P. G. Conard, and A. A. McLean. "Subunit Herpes Simplex Virus-2 Vaccine." In *The Human Herpesviruses: An Interdisciplinary Perspective*, edited by A. J. Nahmias, W. R. Dowdle, and R. F. Schinazi, 504–6. New York: Elsevier, 1981.

Lazar, M. P. "Vaccination for Recurrent Herpes Simplex Infection: Initiation of a New Disease Site Following the Use of Unmodified Material Containing the Live Virus." *Archives of Dermatology* 73 (1956):70–71.

Takahashi, M., T. Otsuka, Y. Okuno, Y. Asano, T. Yazaki, and S. Isomura. "Live Vaccine Used to Prevent the Spread of Varicella in Children in Hospital." *Lancet* 2 (1974):1288–90.

Glossary

Glossary / 181

acquired immunodeficiency syndrome (AIDS). Unexplained and abrupt loss of normal immune function occurring almost exclusively among male homosexuals, intravenous drug addicts, and hemophiliacs. AIDS is probably caused by a human retrovirus.

acute disease. Disease that lasts a short time, usually less than a month.

acyclovir. Trade name Zovirax. Potent antiviral drug that interferes with the reproduction of herpesviruses. Now licensed in ointment and intravenous forms. An oral form is being tested.

AIDS. Acronym for acquired immunodeficiency syndrome.

antibiotic. Substance capable of killing microorganisms, most commonly bacteria.

antibody. Large protein molecule made by B-lymphocytes to fight harmful antagonists such as bacteria, viruses, and cancer cells.

antigen. Substance seen as foreign by the immune system, provoking a response that includes production of antibody, recognition and memory of the invader.

antilymphocyte globulin. Antiserum that destroys lymphocytes in order to protect a transplanted organ.

arildone. Experimental antiviral drug, potentially broad spectrum, with activity against herpes simplex, cytomegalovirus, and polio.

attenuation. Method of vaccine production whereby the vaccine material is manipulated in the laboratory to render it harmless.

autoinoculation. Self-spread of infection from one part of the body to another.

azathioprine. Brand name Imuran. Potent immunosuppressive drug used to prevent rejection of transplanted organs.

bacterium. Microorganism that possesses its own enzymes and reproductive machinery and that can multiply inside and outside host cells. Visible under the light microscope.

B-lymphocyte. Lymphocyte designed to make antibodies against foreign substances.

Burkitt's lymphoma. Malignant tumor of B-lymphocytes.

canker sore. Ulcers inside the mouth that may be recurrent but which are not due to herpes.

chromosome. Strand of DNA, present in the nucleus of every human cell, that carries all heritable information.

chronic disease. Disease lasting a long time, always more than a month.

chronobiology. Science of the effect of time on living systems.

cold sore. Common term for herpes of the lip or herpes labialis.

conjunctiva. Membrane that lines the eyelids and covers the white portions of the eyes. Infection of this membrane is called conjunctivitis.

controlled trial. Clinical test in which one group of subjects is used as a standard of comparison to determine the usefulness of a new medical approach. The control group frequently does not receive any specific therapy and thus represents the natural history (untreated course) of the disease being evaluated.

cornea. Outer clear window of the eye.

cot. Sheath worn to protect a finger during application of medication to an infected area.

cyclosporine. Trade name Sandimmune. Potent new antirejection medicine.

cytarabine. Product name Cytosar-U. Drug useful for treatment of certain cancers but ineffective against human herpesviruses.

cytomegalovirus (CMV). One of the five human herpesviruses. A cause of birth defects, monolike illnesses, and infections in immunosuppressed patients.

cytoplasm. Main portion of the cell, excluding the nucleus.

dendrite. Threadlike extension of a nerve cell. The term also is used to describe the appearance of herpes keratitis.

dermatome. Area of skin supplied by nerve fibers from a single dorsal root ganglion.

DMSO. Acronym for dimethyl sulfoxide. Organic solvent ineffective in treatment of herpesvirus diseases.

DNA. Acronym for deoxyribonucleic acid. Large molecules that contain the genetic code of human cells and also that of many microorganisms including all members of the herpes family.

dorsal root ganglion. One of many collections of nerve cell bodies near the spine that are the site of latency for herpes simplex and varicella-zoster viruses.

double-blind trial. Clinical test in which neither the patients nor the researchers know who is receiving what test substance until the study is concluded.

electroencephalogram. Recording of electrical waves from the brain. Used to diagnose many brain diseases including herpes encephalitis.

encephalitis. Inflammation of the brain most often caused by viruses.

enzyme. Protein capable of changing another substance within the body. Enzymes are used to build up, tear down, or alter the structure of other molecules.

epidemiology. Science of tracing the origins and relationships of factors promoting disease and disease spread.

Epstein-Barr virus (EBV). One of the five members of the human herpes family. Causes infectious mononucleosis.

fever blister. Common term for herpes of the lip or herpes labialis.

first episode. First *symptomatic* infection. The "first" episode is not always our primary (very first) infection because the latter may have been asymptomatic.

ganglion. Collection of nerve cell bodies. A ganglion contains the nuclei of neurons that can harbor latent herpes simplex and varicella-zoster viruses.

gene. Segment of a DNA molecule specifying the production of a single substance.

glaucoma. Increased pressure inside the eye, which, if untreated, can lead to blindness.

glycoprotein. Class of compounds containing proteins and sugar. Located on the outside part of human herpesviruses, glycoproteins are good stimulators of immunity and for this reason are being used to produce subunit vaccines.

gonorrhea. Venereal disease due to the bacterium *Neisseria gonorrhoeae*.

hematology. Medical science specializing in diseases of the blood.

hemodialysis. Method of directly removing poisonous substances from the bloodstream of patients whose kidneys cannot do this for them.

hemophilia. Inherited bleeding disease affecting males primarily, characterized by lack of an essential clotting factor. Bleeding is controlled by giving frequent transfusions containing the missing factor.

herpes. Short for herpes simplex type 1 and type 2, or the diseases they produce.

herpes family. Five human herpesviruses that include herpes simplex type 1, herpes simplex type 2, varicella-zoster virus, Epstein-Barr virus, and cytomegalovirus.

herpes labialis. Herpes of the lips. Also called cold sores and fever blisters.

herpes simiae. Herpesvirus of monkeys that can cause serious disease in humans handling infected animals. Also called herpes B.

herpes simplex type 1. One of the five human herpesviruses. The most common cause of oral herpes.

herpes simplex type 2. One of the five human herpesviruses. The most common cause of genital herpes.

herpes zoster. Synonym for shingles.

herpesvirus. Any member of the herpes family.

herpetic gingivostomatitis. Herpes infection inside the mouth. Often affects both the gums and surrounding mucous membranes.

heterophile titer. Blood test to diagnose infectious mononucleosis.

Hodgkin's disease. Specific form of cancer of the lymph glands and spleen.

idoxuridine. Trade names Stoxil, Herplex, Dendrid. Antiviral drug effective against herpes keratitis but ineffective against other herpetic infections.

immunization. Active immunization means to stimulate the immune system to develop its own defense against foreign invaders. Passive immunization means to receive someone else's immunity usually in the form of globulin or plasma injections.

immunology. Science of host response against potentially harmful substances, especially microorganisms and cancer cells.

immunosuppressed. Referring to persons whose basic medical condition and/or drug therapy has weakened their immune defenses, rendering them highly susceptible to infection.

incidence. Number of cases of a certain disease in a given period.

interferon. Glycoprotein produced by our cells in response to foreign invaders, especially viruses. Interferon preparations are being used experimentally for treatment of viral infections and cancers.

iritis. Infection of the lens of the eye.

Kaposi's sarcoma. Specific form of cancer often found in AIDS patients.

keratitis. Infection of the cornea.

Legionnaires' Disease. Infection characterized by fever and respiratory symptoms due to the bacterium *Legionnella pneumophila*.

lesion. Area of disease in a certain tissue or organ. In this book the term usually refers to sores of the skin or mucous membranes produced by herpesviruses.

leukemia. Cancer of the white blood cells.

leukocyte. White blood cell.

lymph node. Also called lymph gland. Specialized collections of tissue scattered throughout the body that produce lymphocytes and cleanse the lymph fluid received from lymphatic ducts.

lymphocyte. Type of white blood cell. Some lymphocytes produce antibodies; some are programmed to destroy cells; and some have the ability to remember foreign invaders.

lymphocytosis. Elevation in the number of lymphocytes circulating in the bloodstream.

lymphogranuloma venereum (LGV). Venereal disease caused by the microorganism *Chlamydia trachomatis*.

macrophage. White cell, found in the bloodstream and in tissues, whose primary job is to recognize invading substances and process them so that B-lymphocytes can produce antibody against them.

meningitis. Inflammation of the coverings of the brain and spinal cord, most often due to bacteria, but sometimes caused by viruses.

microorganism. Living being too small to be seen by the naked eye. Examples include bacteria, fungi, and viruses.

mucous membranes. Soft tissue that lines the inside of our nose, mouth, gastrointestinal, urinary and genital tracts.

nasopharyngeal carcinoma. Cancer of the nose and throat that has been associated with Epstein-Barr virus.

neonatal herpes. Herpes infection in an infant less than one month old.

neonatologist. Pediatrician specializing in diseases of premature and newborn infants.

neuron. A cell that conducts nerve signals to and from their site of origin.

nucleus. Spherical body within the cell that contains specialized structures including the chromosomes.

opportunistic infection. Infection due to a microorganism that causes disease only in immunosuppressed persons.

oral herpes. Herpes simplex infection of the lips and/or mouth.

paresthesia. Abnormal sensation such as feeling heat when you are not touching a hot object.

pathology. Medical science specializing in recognition of diseases by examination of organs and tissues. Pathology also designates the damage a specific disease causes a human being.

photophobia. Abnormal intolerance to light.

postherpetic neuralgia. Chronic pain that occasionally follows an acute shingles attack.

prednisone. Immunosuppressive steroid given to treat certain cancers and to prevent rejection of a transplanted organ.

prevalence. Frequency of a condition. In contrast with incidence, prevalence does not have a time denominator. In other words, if 10 people in a 100-member community have a disease today, the prevalence is 10 percent.

primary infection. The very first infection with a particular virus. Primary infections may or may not be symptomatic.

prodrome. Symptom that heralds the beginning of a disease.

prophylaxis. Method of disease prevention.

prospective study. Study that accepts patients before or at the beginning of a disease process and follows them for a specified period.

reactivation. Reawakening of virus latent in the body.

recombinant DNA technology. Commonly referred to as gene splicing, this powerful approach utilizes one microorganism to reproduce the genes or gene products of another.

recurrence. Infection caused by a microorganism that has infected us in the past. A recurrence may be due to reactivation or reinfection.

reinfection. Reintroduction from an outside source of a microorganism that has infected us previously.

rejection. Our natural immune response against foreign tissue, resulting in damage to or destruction of a transplanted organ.

remission. The period when a disease (especially cancer) is inapparent but not necessarily cured.

resistance. Condition whereby a microorganism learns to defy a previously effective antibacterial or antiviral drug.

retrospective study. Study in which patients are analyzed after they have experienced the disease under investigation.

Reye syndrome. Disease that suddenly attacks the liver and brain. The basic cause is unknown, but Reye syndrome is often preceded by certain viral infections, especially influenza B and chickenpox. An association has been made between taking aspirin and Reye syndrome.

ribavirin. Experimental antiviral drug that provided beneficial results against genital herpes in one study. May also be effective against respiratory viruses including influenza.

shedding. Term used by virologists to indicate active multiplication of viruses, inferring that live viruses are freely present in bodily secretions or skin lesions.

steroids. Class of hormones that decreases inflammation but also produces immunosuppression.

subunit vaccine. Vaccine made from a part of the whole microorganism.

symptomatic. Sick. Symptomatic patients recognize they have a disease because they are experiencing specific physical problems.

syndrome. Group of signs and symptoms characterizing a specific disease.

syphilis. Venereal disease due to the bacterium *Treponema pallidum*.

therapeutic index. Ratio of effectiveness of a drug versus its side effects. A drug with a good therapeutic index would be highly effective for the disease being treated without producing any adverse effects.

thymidine kinase. Enzyme induced in cells infected by herpes simplex and varicella-zoster virus. Presence of this special enzyme in the infected cells activates certain antiviral drugs, such as acyclovir.

tissue culture. Technique of cultivating living cells outside their natural host.

Tissue cultures are used to grow viruses, just as liquid artificial media are used to grow bacteria.

T-lymphocyte. Class of lymphocytes that can recognize foreign invaders, remember them, and specifically destroy cancerous or infected cells. T-lymphocytes do not produce antibodies but may be aided and abetted by antibodies.

tolerance. Situation in which the body becomes inured to a particular drug and no longer responds to it. This pertains especially to narcotics.

toxin. Poison. Substance detrimental to normal cells.

transfer factor. Protein prepared from lymphocytes of an immune donor that when injected makes the recipient's lymphocytes immune to a certain virus or cancer for a short time.

trifluorothymidine. Brand name Viroptic. Antiviral drug effective against herpes keratitis.

trigeminal. Referring to the fifth cranial nerve or its ganglion. The trigeminal ganglion frequently is the site of latency for herpes simplex type 1.

Tzanck test. Procedure to detect herpesvirus infections by directly examining blister scrapings.

ulcer. Lesion characterized by loss of normal surface, creating a shallow, painful crater.

urethra. Mucous membrane tube that permits us to expel urine from the bladder. The urethra frequently is damaged in genital herpes infections, making urination painful.

vaccine. Suspension of microorganisms, or their products, that when inoculated into a recipient confers protection against disease produced by the natural form of that microorganism.

vaccinia. Virus of cowpox inoculated into human beings to prevent smallpox. The words *vaccine* and *vaccination* are derived from this first viral vaccine.

vaginitis. Infection of the female birth canal.

varicella-zoster virus. One of the five members of the human herpes family. Cause of chickenpox and shingles.

vesicle. Blister.

vidarabine. Trade name Vira-A. Formerly known as adenine arabinoside or ara-A. Antiviral drug effective against certain herpes simplex and varicella-zoster virus infections. Both intravenous and eye preparations are licensed.

virion. Complete virus particle.

virus. Tiny microorganism, visible under the electron microscope, that is capable of reproducing only inside living cells.

whitlow. Small abscesses of the fingers or hands caused by herpes simplex virus.

zoster. Synonym for shingles.

Index